T0263324

Podiatric Dermatology

Editor

TRACEY C. VLAHOVIC

CLINICS IN PODIATRIC MEDICINE AND SURGERY

www.podiatric.theclinics.com

Consulting Editor
THOMAS J. CHANG

October 2021 • Volume 38 • Number 4

ELSEVIER

1600 John F. Kennedy Boulevard • Suite 1800 • Philadelphia, Pennsylvania, 19103-2899

http://www.theclinics.com

CLINICS IN PODIATRIC MEDICINE AND SURGERY Volume 38, Number 4
October 2021 ISSN 0891-8422, ISBN-13: 978-0-323-98771-4

Editor: Lauren Boyle
Developmental Editor: Diana Grace Ang

© 2021 Elsevier Inc. All rights reserved.

This periodical and the individual contributions contained in it are protected under copyright by Elsevier, and the following terms and conditions apply to their use:

Photocopying
Single photocopies of single articles may be made for personal use as allowed by national copyright laws. Permission of the Publisher and payment of a fee is required for all other photocopying, including multiple or systematic copying, copying for advertising or promotional purposes, resale, and all forms of document delivery. Special rates are available for educational institutions that wish to make photocopies for non-profit educational classroom use. For information on how to seek permission visit www.elsevier.com/permissions or call: (+44) 1865 843830 (UK)/(+1) 215 239 3804 (USA).

Derivative Works
Subscribers may reproduce tables of contents or prepare lists of articles including abstracts for internal circulation within their institutions. Permission of the Publisher is required for resale or distribution outside the institution. Permission of the Publisher is required for all other derivative works, including compilations and translations (please consult www.elsevier.com/permissions).

Electronic Storage or Usage
Permission of the Publisher is required to store or use electronically any material contained in this periodical, including any article or part of an article (please consult www.elsevier.com/permissions). Except as outlined above, no part of this publication may be reproduced, stored in a retrieval system or transmitted in any form or by any means, electronic, mechanical, photocopying, recording or otherwise, without prior written permission of the Publisher.

Notice
No responsibility is assumed by the Publisher for any injury and/or damage to persons or property as a matter of products liability, negligence or otherwise, or from any use or operation of any methods, products, instructions or ideas contained in the material herein. Because of rapid advances in the medical sciences, in particular, independent verification of diagnoses and drug dosages should be made.

Although all advertising material is expected to conform to ethical (medical) standards, inclusion in this publication does not constitute a guarantee or endorsement of the quality or value of such product or of the claims made of it by its manufacturer.

Clinics in Podiatric Medicine and Surgery (ISSN 0891-8422) is published quarterly by Elsevier Inc., 360 Park Avenue South, New York, NY 10010-1710. Months of issue are January, April, July, and October. Business and Editorial Offices: 1600 John F. Kennedy Blvd., Ste. 1800, Philadelphia, PA 19103-2899. Customer Service Office: 3251 Riverport Lane, Maryland Heights, MO 63043. Periodicals postage paid at New York, NY and additional mailing offices. Subscription prices are $310.00 per year for US individuals, $750.00 per year for US institutions, $100.00 per year for US students and residents, $382.00 per year for Canadian individuals, $776.00 for Canadian institutions, $462.00 for international individuals, $776.00 per year for international institutions, $100.00 per year for Canadian students/residents, and $220.00 per year for foreign students/residents. To receive student/resident rate, orders must be accompanied by name of affiliated institution, date of term, and the *signature* of program/residency coordinator on institution letterhead. Orders will be billed at individual rate until proof of status is received. Foreign air speed delivery is included in all *Clinics* subscription prices. All prices are subject to change without notice. POSTMASTER: Send address changes to *Clinics in Podiatric Medicine and Surgery*, Elsevier Health Sciences Division, Subscription Customer Service, 3251 Riverport Lane, Maryland Heights, MO 63043. **Customer Service: 1-800-654-2452 (US). From outside of the US, call 314-447-8871. Fax: 314-447-8029. E-mail: JournalsCustomerService-usa@elsevier.com (for print support); JournalsOnlineSupport-usa@elsevier.com (for online support).**

Reprints. For copies of 100 or more of articles in this publication, please contact the Commercial Reprints Department, Elsevier Inc., 360 Park Avenue South, New York, NY 10010-1710. Tel.: 212-633-3874; Fax: 212-633-3820; E-mail: reprints@elsevier.com.

Clinics in Podiatric Medicine and Surgery is covered in *MEDLINE/PubMed (Index Medicus)* and *EMBASE/Excerpta Medica*.

Contributors

CONSULTING EDITOR

THOMAS J. CHANG, DPM
Clinical Professor and Past Chairman, Department of Podiatric Surgery, California College of Podiatric Medicine, Faculty, The Podiatry Institute, Redwood Orthopedic Surgery Associates, Santa Rosa, California

EDITOR

TRACEY C. VLAHOVIC, DPM, FFPM, RCPS (Glasg)
Clinical Professor, Department of Podiatric Medicine, Temple University School of Podiatric Medicine, Philadelphia, Pennsylvania

AUTHORS

ADAM ABBOUD, DPM
Temple University School of Podiatric Medicine, Philadelphia, Pennsylvania

VICTORIA ADENIRAN, DPM
Temple University School of Podiatric Medicine, Philadelphia, Pennsylvania

MICHAEL AN, DPM
Temple University School of Podiatric Medicine, Philadelphia, Pennsylvania

MADELEINE BARBE, DPM
Temple University School of Podiatric Medicine, Philadelphia, Pennsylvania

ANDREA BATRA, DPM
Temple University School of Podiatric Medicine, Philadelphia, Pennsylvania

ADAM BHATTI, DPM
Temple University School of Podiatric Medicine, Philadelphia, Pennsylvania

GARRETT BIELA, DPM
Temple University School of Podiatric Medicine, Philadelphia, Pennsylvania

LEV BLEKHER, DPM
Temple University School of Podiatric Medicine, Philadelphia, Pennsylvania

JARED BLUM, DPM
Temple University School of Podiatric Medicine, Philadelphia, Pennsylvania

MICHAEL BROWN, DPM
Temple University School of Podiatric Medicine, Philadelphia, Pennsylvania

SHELBY BUSCH, DPM
Temple University School of Podiatric Medicine, Philadelphia, Pennsylvania

ZARNAB BUTTA, DPM
Temple University School of Podiatric Medicine, Philadelphia, Pennsylvania

CORINNA CASTILLO, DPM
Temple University School of Podiatric Medicine, Philadelphia, Pennsylvania

ASHER CHERIAN, DPM
Temple University School of Podiatric Medicine, Philadelphia, Pennsylvania

JIN O. CHO, DPM
Temple University School of Podiatric Medicine, Philadelphia, Pennsylvania

SAAKSHI CHOWDHARY, DPM
Temple University School of Podiatric Medicine, Philadelphia, Pennsylvania

SALIL DESAI, DPM
Temple University School of Podiatric Medicine, Philadelphia, Pennsylvania

MARCUS DUVAL, DPM
Temple University School of Podiatric Medicine, Philadelphia, Pennsylvania

JOSH EKLADIOS, DPM
Temple University School of Podiatric Medicine, Philadelphia, Pennsylvania

KALEN FARR, DPM
Temple University School of Podiatric Medicine, Philadelphia, Pennsylvania

CIESCO FEBRIAN, DPM
Temple University School of Podiatric Medicine, Philadelphia, Pennsylvania

THOMAS FERRISE, DPM
Temple University School of Podiatric Medicine, Philadelphia, Pennsylvania

FLAVIA FILISIO, DPM
Temple University School of Podiatric Medicine, Philadelphia, Pennsylvania

MICHELLE GARCIA, DPM
Temple University School of Podiatric Medicine, Philadelphia, Pennsylvania

STEPHANIE GOLDING, DPM
Temple University School of Podiatric Medicine, Philadelphia, Pennsylvania

SAM GORELIK, DPM
Temple University School of Podiatric Medicine, Philadelphia, Pennsylvania

NAGA GOVARDHANAM, DPM
Temple University School of Podiatric Medicine, Philadelphia, Pennsylvania

OLIVIA HAMMOND, DPM
Temple University School of Podiatric Medicine, Philadelphia, Pennsylvania

JACQUELINE C. HIGGINS, DPM
Temple University School of Podiatric Medicine, Philadelphia, Pennsylvania

RUSSELL HILL, DPM
Temple University School of Podiatric Medicine, Philadelphia, Pennsylvania

JASON JOLLIFFE, DPM
Temple University School of Podiatric Medicine, Philadelphia, Pennsylvania

SUSHILA KABADI, DPM
Temple University School of Podiatric Medicine, Philadelphia, Pennsylvania

KUSHKARAN KAUR, DPM
Temple University School of Podiatric Medicine, Philadelphia, Pennsylvania

EUI T. KIM, DPM
Temple University School of Podiatric Medicine, Philadelphia, Pennsylvania

AMIDA KUAH, DPM
Temple University School of Podiatric Medicine, Philadelphia, Pennsylvania

NISHANI KURUPPU, DPM
Temple University School of Podiatric Medicine, Philadelphia, Pennsylvania

RYAN LAZAR, DPM
Temple University School of Podiatric Medicine, Philadelphia, Pennsylvania

ALEXANDER LEOS, DPM
Temple University School of Podiatric Medicine, Philadelphia, Pennsylvania

ELIZABETH FERBER LINDVIG, DPM
Temple University School of Podiatric Medicine, Philadelphia, Pennsylvania

MENG LIU, DPM
Temple University School of Podiatric Medicine, Philadelphia, Pennsylvania

MICHAEL F. MASI, DPM
Temple University School of Podiatric Medicine, Philadelphia, Pennsylvania

AUSTIN MISHKO, DPM
Temple University School of Podiatric Medicine, Philadelphia, Pennsylvania

AHMAD NAMOUS, DPM
Temple University School of Podiatric Medicine, Philadelphia, Pennsylvania

AMBER O'CONNOR, DPM
Temple University School of Podiatric Medicine, Philadelphia, Pennsylvania

ALEXANDRU ONICA, DPM
Temple University School of Podiatric Medicine, Philadelphia, Pennsylvania

SHALIN PANCHIGAR, DPM
Temple University School of Podiatric Medicine, Philadelphia, Pennsylvania

ALEXANDRA PARISH, DPM
Temple University School of Podiatric Medicine, Philadelphia, Pennsylvania

KARI PHAN, DPM
Temple University School of Podiatric Medicine, Philadelphia, Pennsylvania

MATTHEW PITRE, DPM
Temple University School of Podiatric Medicine, Philadelphia, Pennsylvania

RAFAY QURESHI, DPM
Temple University School of Podiatric Medicine, Philadelphia, Pennsylvania

MICHAEL ROMANI, DPM
Temple University School of Podiatric Medicine, Philadelphia, Pennsylvania

RYAN SHANER, DPM
Temple University School of Podiatric Medicine, Philadelphia, Pennsylvania

ALEX SHELTZER, DPM
Temple University School of Podiatric Medicine, Philadelphia, Pennsylvania

ANKITA SHETE, DPM
Temple University School of Podiatric Medicine, Philadelphia, Pennsylvania

DARYL SILVA, DPM
Temple University School of Podiatric Medicine, Philadelphia, Pennsylvania

TYMOTEUSZ SIWY, DPM
Temple University School of Podiatric Medicine, Philadelphia, Pennsylvania

ALEX SPEER, DPM
Temple University School of Podiatric Medicine, Philadelphia, Pennsylvania

BENTON STEWART, DPM
Temple University School of Podiatric Medicine, Philadelphia, Pennsylvania

HEATHER TRAN, DPM
Temple University School of Podiatric Medicine, Philadelphia, Pennsylvania

SON TRAN, DPM
Temple University School of Podiatric Medicine, Philadelphia, Pennsylvania

YAAKOV TROPPER, DPM
Temple University School of Podiatric Medicine, Philadelphia, Pennsylvania

VICTORIA TROVILLION, DPM
Temple University School of Podiatric Medicine, Philadelphia, Pennsylvania

CAROLINA LORDELO VAN PELT, DPM
Temple University School of Podiatric Medicine, Philadelphia, Pennsylvania

TRACEY C. VLAHOVIC, DPM, FFPM, RCPS (Glasg)
Clinical Professor, Department of Podiatric Medicine, Temple University School of
Podiatric Medicine, Philadelphia, Pennsylvania

SONYA WALI, DPM
Temple University School of Podiatric Medicine, Philadelphia, Pennsylvania

JASON WELLNER, DPM,
Temple University School of Podiatric Medicine, Philadelphia, Pennsylvania

DELANEY J. H. WICKRAMAGE, DPM
Temple University School of Podiatric Medicine, Philadelphia, Pennsylvania

KEVIN WOTRING, BS
Medical Student Year 4, Temple University School of Podiatric Medicine, Philadelphia,
Pennsylvania

KAYLA WRIGHT, DPM
Temple University School of Podiatric Medicine, Philadelphia, Pennsylvania

Contents

Onychomycosis is one of the most frequent nail pathologies in podiatry practices. Differential diagnoses with the clinical presentation may delay an accurate diagnosis and timely treatment. This article discusses the technique and benefits of using a dermatoscope to improve patient care of this common disorder.

Traditionally, plantar warts or verrucae are often diagnosed by visual appearance and the lateral squeeze test. At times, these methods are not able to elucidate the difference between a plantar wart and a callus. The use of the dermatoscope can not only distinguish the difference between a wart and a callus, which ultimately helps to customize treatment plans to increase efficacy, but also be used to follow the therapeutic effects of treatment. The dermatoscope is a tool that can be used in the diagnosis of plantar verrucae and in assessment of the success of therapy.

Disappearing nail bed (DNB) is a condition characterized by irreversible epithelialization of the nail bed following long-standing onycholysis. This phenomenon can occur in fingernails and toenails. Factors implicated in the development of DNB include trauma, manicuring, and onychotillomania and dermatologic conditions like psoriasis and dermatitis. Specifically for the toenail, contributing factors also include increasing age, history of trauma, surgery, onychomycosis, and onychogryphosis. A grading system that stages the progression of onycholysis to DNB has been proposed to aid clinicians in the diagnosis and treatment of these conditions. Several methods have been designated for the treatment of DNB.

> Recent studies have shown that a superficial fungal infection such as onychomycosis may form complex biofilms. Although most individuals susceptible to documented fungal biofilm infections are immunocompromised, physical damage to the nail or concurrent infection with other organisms is also a common risk factor in developing nail biofilm. The complex nature of the biofilm, which includes efflux pumps and the formation of a virulent extracellular matrix, helps it evade the immune system. Although there is no standardized treatment for fungal biofilms in onychomycosis, various studies using antimicrobials and lasers have shown some efficacy in treating human fingernails.

> The chemical composition and thickness of nails are obstacles for treatments of various nail diseases, such as onychomycosis. Topical medications are currently the preferred method of treatment because of reduced adverse systemic effects. However, penetration of the product from the nail plate into the nail bed continues to be an issue because of factors such as distance required to reach the target area, chemical barriers, and drug inactivation upon keratin binding. Beyond developing novel drugs, some studies have investigated mechanical and chemical methods to optimize drug delivery. The issue of nail diseases is still a challenge and requires multifactorial treatments.

> Plantar psoriasis negatively affects the quality of life for patients due to its weight-bearing location. Most therapeutic studies for psoriasis focus on total body surface changes and rarely report specific effects of the plantar and palmar areas. This review focuses on therapeutic options for plantar psoriasis ranging from topical therapy to phototherapy to biological therapy. Treatment should be approached as a stepwise gradient beginning with topicals and progressing to systemics. As always, review of the patient's severity of condition, health status, and impact on quality of life is needed to individualize therapy for the best patient care.

> Psoriasis is a common inflammatory disorder with potentially severe systemic and dermatologic consequences. As traditional treatments for this condition fail, biologics are emerging as the next promising therapy for moderate-to-severe cases, especially for the lower extremity. This review examines current research on monoclonal antibodies that target specific

cytokines including interleukin-23 (IL-23), IL-12, tumor necrosis factor alpha, and IL-17 involved in pathologic inflammatory processes.

Melanoma accounts for more than 100,000 new cancer cases each year, and a minority (3%–15%) involve the foot and ankle. Case studies and isolated data set analyses report infrequent plantar melanomas, with these tumors more commonly encountered in non-whites. The absolute incidence of plantar melanoma is approximately the same in all races, but it is a more common type of cutaneous melanoma in non-white populations. Plantar melanoma is more prevalent in women, potentially a result of increased inflammation from uncomfortable shoes. When presenting on the plantar surface of the foot, features atypical of classic cutaneous melanoma are often present.

CLINICS IN PODIATRIC MEDICINE AND SURGERY

SERIES OF RELATED INTEREST

Orthopedic Clinics
https://www.orthopedic.theclinics.com/
Clinics in Sports Medicine
https://www.sportsmed.theclinics.com/
Foot and Ankle Clinics
https://www.foot.theclinics.com/
Physical Medicine and Rehabilitation Clinics
https://www.pmr.theclinics.com/

THE CLINICS ARE AVAILABLE ONLINE!
Access your subscription at:
www.theclinics.com

Foreword

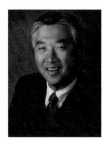

Thomas J. Chang, DPM
Consulting Editor

Speaking personally, Dermatology continues to be a challenging area to gain knowledge and confidence in my clinical practice. As a student at PCPM, we were all impressed when Dr Harvey Lemont would come into clinic and make an instant diagnosis of skin conditions from the doorway. Over the past decades, I have appreciated and benefited from occasional dermatologic exposure from Dr Gary Dockery, Dr Mary Crawford, and Dr Brad Bakotic. They have enhanced our knowledge of Podiatric Dermatology in countless lectures, hands-on workshops, and written publications.

Currently, in the area of Podiatric Medicine and Dermatology, Dr Tracey Vlahovic has established her reputation as a tremendous educator and respected author on numerous articles. I know she has dedicated her career to research in this area, and she has a genuine passion to share her knowledge with the entire foot and ankle community.

These articles have been carefully selected to bring a high level of practicality to our dermatology knowledge base. We will all be more well-rounded physicians of the foot and ankle after reading these works. It is my hope any lower-extremity physician will glean relevant information from each article and find applicability in their clinical practices.

I want to extend my gratitude to Dr Vlahovic and her team for bringing this issue to us.

Thomas J. Chang, DPM
Redwood Orthopedic Surgery Associates
208 Concourse Boulevard
Santa Rosa, CA 95403, USA

E-mail address:
thomaschang14@comcast.net

Clin Podiatr Med Surg 38 (2021) xiii
https://doi.org/10.1016/j.cpm.2021.07.001
0891-8422/21/© 2021 Published by Elsevier Inc.

podiatric.theclinics.com

Preface

Podiatric Dermatology for the Practicing Podiatric Physician

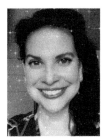

Tracey C. Vlahovic, DPM, FFPM, RCPS (Glasg)
Editor

I am pleased to present a wide range of podiatric dermatology topics that should prove useful to the physician in practice. From dermoscopy of the nails to plantar melanoma, these articles provide the latest information for the practitioner to make evidenced-based choices for patients. Podiatric dermatology is my passion in this profession, and it has always been my goal to give back to my profession with the experience and knowledge I have gained over the years. That said, as a challenge to my students, I encouraged them to critically analyze the literature and write reviews of the topics that are relevant to podiatric medicine. All articles in this issue were written by my former students, who I am now proud to call my colleagues. It truly is my honor to present the work of Temple University School of Podiatric Medicine alumni, and I hope this encourages them and other young podiatric physicians to participate in future article writing and publishing.

Some topics may be new, like disappearing nail bed, but after reading that article, you will realize how often that condition is seen in practice. Dermoscopy may not be a tool you currently use in your practice, but after you read the articles on nails and warts, I hope that it inspires you to delve further into this useful modality that I have found to be indispensable in my practice. Biofilms in the nail unit, I predict, will become a hot topic in future research, but in the meantime, I encourage you to consider how complex the nail unit is for a topical to penetrate to manage onychomycosis. I see patients with psoriasis daily followed by those with shoe dermatitis and want the podiatric clinician to consider other differential diagnoses of skin rashes beyond a fungal origin. For those who manage wound care patients, there are articles on skin manifestations of patients with diabetes, lymphedema therapy, and pyoderma gangrenosum. Last, the article on plantar melanoma should keep this entity as a differential diagnosis when unusual lesions and wounds on the foot appear.

Clin Podiatr Med Surg 38 (2021) xv–xvi
https://doi.org/10.1016/j.cpm.2021.06.013
0891-8422/21/© 2021 Published by Elsevier Inc.

podiatric.theclinics.com

It is my hope that these articles will serve the podiatric physician well and encourage further investigation to provide the highest level of care to our patients presenting with lower-extremity skin concerns.

Tracey C. Vlahovic, DPM, FFPM, RCPS (Glasg)
Department of Podiatric Medicine
Temple University School of Podiatric Medicine
148 North 8th Street
Philadelphia, PA 19107, USA

E-mail address:
traceyv@temple.edu

Dermoscopy of Onychomycosis for the Podiatrist

Tracey C. Vlahovic, DPM, FFPM RCPS (Glasg)*, Michelle Garcia, DPM,
Kevin Wotring, BS

KEYWORDS

- Dermoscopy • Dermatoscope • Onychomycosis • Dystrophic nail

KEY POINTS

- A dermatoscope is a tool that allows one to both provide a visual diagnosis and formulate a stronger differential diagnosis while waiting for the fungal test results to return.
- Noncontact polarized light dermoscopy is often used for the toenails.
- Dermoscopy cannot substitute for mycological testing but it can provide definite insight into nail disease, which allows for initiation of a treatment plan.

INTRODUCTION

Podiatric physicians feel confident in diagnosing toenail onychomycosis clinically due to the vast number of cases seen daily in the office. However, one may have second thoughts about that ability or feel frustrated by the lack of clinical correlation after the return of a few negative clinical laboratory tests such as periodic acid Schiff stain (PAS), KOH and fungal culture, or polymerase chain reaction (PCR) testing. Explanations for a negative fungal test might include where the area of the nail unit that was sampled (nail plate vs nail bed) and its influence on the chosen test as well as the numerous differential diagnoses that are visually identical to onychomycosis. A dermatoscope is a tool that allows one to both provide a visual diagnosis and formulate a stronger differential diagnosis while waiting for the fungal test results to return.

Dermoscopy, or the use of a device that provides noninvasive handheld imaging, was originally intended to assess pigmented lesions on the skin to determine the need for potential biopsy. Over the years, dermatologists have used dermoscopy in

Conflict of Interest: none of the authors have any financial interests to disclose for this article.
Temple University School of Podiatric Medicine, 148 North 8th Street, Philadelphia, PA 19107, USA
* Corresponding author.
E-mail address: traceyv@temple.edu

areas beyond assessing pigmented lesions such as diagnosing inflammatory skin disorders, hair issues, and nail disease. Onychomycosis constitutes 50% of the nail disease that physicians see in the office; therefore, having a device that takes some of the guesswork out of the equation is practical and cost-efficient.[1]

From the clinical perspective, the average dystrophic nail may visually be equivalent to onychomycosis, but a different world emerges with the use of a dermatoscope. For instance, dermoscopy can assist in determining if the nail dystrophy is trauma related (eg, a sport that has hard stops such as basketball), surface staining from nail polish or a sock dye, or even a benign nail matrix tumor known as an onychomatricoma.

In general, the clinical characteristics of onychomycosis include yellow to white to brown discoloration (chromonychia), onycholysis (separation of the nail bed from the nail plate), subungual debris, geographic disturbances of the nail plate surface (Beau lines, onychorrhexis, pitting), brittleness, and subungual hematoma. These findings are not unique to onychomycosis and can appear in other nail pathologies. When the clinician uses a dermatoscope, he or she can magnify these findings, which provides a rapid way to confirm suspicion of onychomycosis and pursue subsequent clinical laboratory testing to ensure the correct diagnosis.

Most dermatoscopes are pocket-sized and can be attached to a smartphone to take photos. However, as the nail plate is a convex surface, it may cause a learning curve for the practitioner to apply the dermatoscope to the nail and obtain the focus of the pathology.

To visualize the nail plate clearly, the dermatoscope is applied to a dry nail without contacting the surface directly. However, if the distal nail edge or the proximal nail fold needs to be examined, ultrasound gel or hand sanitizer is applied as an interface between the nail and the scope to visualize deeper structures. The common pocket dermatoscope provides 10x magnification and is considered a "hybrid" if it has both polarized light and nonpolarized light illumination capabilities. This hybrid scope allows the practitioner to use an interface gel if desired or provides noncontact dermoscopy (**Fig. 1**).

Noncontact polarized light dermoscopy is used for the toenails. The scope is applied about 1 to 2 cm above the area in question and then the examiner places the eye a few centimeters above the scope until the field appears in focus. The distal nail plate in addition to the dorsal nail plate should also be examined. For example, the longitudinal white lines that is often seen with onychomycosis on the dorsal surface of the nail plate can provide confirmation (when you view them from the distal nail) that a benign tumor from the nail matrix is present called an onychomatricoma.

DERMATOSCOPIC FINDINGS OF ONYCHOMYCOSIS

Various investigators have correlated onychomycosis-related patterns with the dermatoscope and a positive fungal test (KOH, culture, PAS, Gomori methenamine silver). For the purposes of this article, distal subungual onychomycosis dermoscopy findings are discussed, as that is the most frequent type of onychomycosis seen.

Piraccini and colleagues were the first to describe the patterns of distal subungual onychomycosis in comparison to traumatic onycholysis via dermoscopy.[2] Because traumatic onycholysis and onychomycosis can be virtually impossible to distinguish without mycological tests, this study aimed to define the dermatoscopic characteristics of the 57 patients who had dermoscopy, clinical photography, and mycological testing (KOH and culture) of their affected great toenail. For distal subungual onychomycosis specimens, the most specific dermatoscopic patterns that the study investigators saw were the "jagged edge with spikes" and "longitudinal striae."

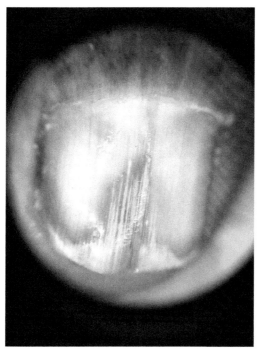

Fig. 1. Dermoscopy of DSO showing yellow streaks directed to proximal nail fold. DSO, distal subungual onychomycosis.

The jagged edge with spikes pattern describes a serrated knifelike edge appearance of white streaks at the tip of the onycholysis pointing toward the proximal nail fold. Longitudinal striae are white to yellow fingerlike projections that also point toward the proximal nail. The study investigators also reported blackish globules that were subungual hemorrhages in nails with distal subungual onychomycosis, but this finding was not as specific as the 2 previously mentioned patterns.[2] They were also the first to coin the "aurora" pattern term, which describes the pigmentation produced in linear figures reminiscent of the aurora borealis phenomenon. In comparison to the distal subungual onychomycotic nails, the investigators noted linear edges of white discoloration in specific traumatic onycholysis 100% of the time[2] (**Fig. 2**).

Kaynak and team reported the frequency of dermatoscopic findings in onychomycosis that were confirmed to be distal subungual onychomycosis by either PAS or hematoxylin and eosin stain/fungal culture in 97 patients.[3] Unlike the work by Piraccini and colleagues, Kaynak and coworkers did not observe as high a frequency of the jagged edge pattern. Their laboratory confirmation of the following patterns seen with the dermatoscope yielded a high diagnostic sensitivity of distal subungual onychomycosis. "The ruin appearance" and various manifestations of leukonychia were their highest-rated dermatoscopic patterns that correlated to distal subungual onychomycosis. The ruin appearance describes the visual appearance of the subungual debris and its ability to affect the underside of the nail plate.

Subungual debris is the skin's inflammatory reaction pattern to the process of fungal invasion. One can best view this by positioning the dermatoscope at the distal edge of the nail plate. Leukonychia or white discoloration may appear on the nail plate in punctate (spots), homogeneous (discrete areas), or as a longitudinal (thin streaks) fashion.

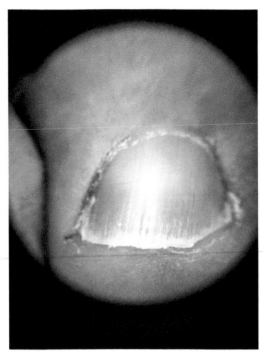

Fig. 2. Dermoscopy of DSO showing onycholysis with the uneven longitudinal streaks.

These patterns are thought to correlate with the presence of the fungus in the ventral surface of the nail plate. In addition, Kaynak and colleagues observed the distal irregular termination pattern, which presents as an irregular and crumbly nail plate edge at the hyponychium.[3] Although one can obviously see this clinically, a dermatoscopic view gives the clinician a whole new appreciation for the dryness and brittleness of the nail plate distally.

The findings of Yorulmaz and Yalcin, who only used KOH as their means of mycologic testing, correlated with the findings of the studies of Piraccini and Kaynak.[2–4] Their study of 81 patients with onychomycosis had consistent patterns of jagged edges with spikes, longitudinal streaks, subungual hyperkeratosis (ruin appearance), and leukonychia. The consistent longitudinal patterns speak to the anatomy of the nail unit. The nail plate has longitudinal rete ridges that fit into the ridges of the nail bed.[4] In distal subungual onychomycosis, the fungal invasion advances from the hyponychium distally and travels proximally. The hyponychium serves as a weak barrier between the world and the nail unit, which dermatophytes exploit. The weak adhesions at the hyponychium are of little concern, as the fungus metabolizes keratin and colonizes the nail unit while following the linear pattern created by the longitudinal rete ridges.[4]

Practitioners can also visualize another anomaly of onychomycosis, the dermatophytoma, both clinically and via the dermatoscope. A dermatophytoma is an amalgamation of hyphae and scales and appears as a distinct yellow to brown digitation in the nail plate.[5] With the dermatoscope, the dermatophytoma appears as a "homogeneous, matte, yellow-orange discoloration" subungually and connects to the distal margin of the nail by a linear yellow-white band.[5]

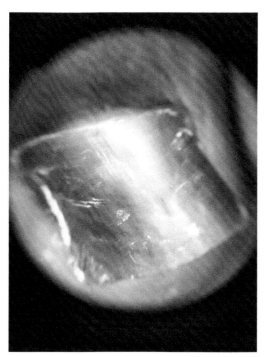

Fig. 3. Dermoscopy of DSO showing chromomycosis and a linear black lesion centrally (subungual hematoma).

The dermatoscopic patterns of distal subungual onychomycosis help to determine which nails to sample for mycologic testing. Once one or more of the patterns described earlier have been observed, the lead investigator focuses on that nail to retrieve as much proximal subungual debris as possible to provide a better sample for fungal culture or PAS, PCR, and so on.

As mentioned earlier, traumatic onycholysis yielded a linear edge pattern in comparison to the jagged or digitated edge of distal subungual onychomycosis, which is often surrounded by a pale-pink nail bed.[5] Beyond traumatic onycholysis, if the practitioner suspects a psoriatic nail, he or she will notice an erythematous border at the edge of detachment or onycholysis as well as a yellow discoloration.[5] When working up nail issues as a result of an inflammatory skin issue, the practitioner may also use the dermatoscope on the hyponychium and even the proximal nail fold. With psoriatic nails, dermoscopy of the hyponychium will reveal an irregular and dilated capillary pattern.[5] Dermoscopy will also show onychorrhexis and Beau lines clearly as well as superficial staining that may result from nail polish or socks.

Dermoscopy can be used to confirm that a nail attached to a hammertoe or mallet toe is truly dystrophic versus onychomycotic. In these cases, the nail will be devoid of the patterns for distal subungual onychomycosis but will have significant Beau lines or onychorrhexis due to the chronic repetitive trauma from the pathomechanics involved.

Dermoscopy will also allow the practitioner to differentiate a subungual hematoma from onychomycosis.[5] The dark discoloration one sees in onychomycosis clinically may be fungal melanonychia or an accumulation of subungual blood. Subungual hematoma is the most common cause of brown-black discoloration in the nails and is often a result of chronic repetitive trauma from shoes or direct injury. A true subungual

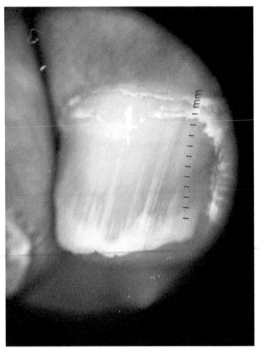

Fig. 5. Dermoscopy of DSO showing longitudinal striae directing toward the proximal nail fold.

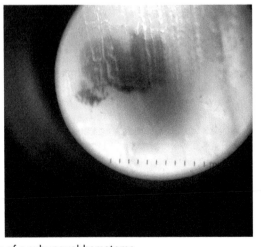

Fig. 4. Dermoscopy of a subungual hematoma.

hematoma will show a round area with small dots or globules at the edges of the lesion[5] (**Figs. 3–5**).

SUMMARY

Dermoscopy of the nail unit provides a simple and efficient technique to define a diagnosis. The reason for highlighting the distinctive features of distal subungual onychomycosis through dermoscopy is to increase diagnostic accuracy at the point of care while waiting for the mycological test results. Ultimately, dermoscopy cannot substitute for mycological testing but it can provide definite insight into nail disease, which allows for initiation of a treatment plan.

For the patients who prefer topical therapy, dermoscopy of the nail unit may reduce diagnostic delay.[6] For those who prefer oral antifungal therapy, dermoscopy can provide a diagnostic tool that can direct specimen collection for mycology and refinement of a differential diagnosis.

Overall, dermoscopy is a useful tool that should be used more in the podiatric profession, given the amount of nail cases most practitioners see on a weekly basis. After a bit of a learning curve, time, and practice, the podiatric physician should be able to assess a nail efficiently and accurately with the dermatoscope, which ultimately will benefit the patient's care.

CLINICS CARE POINTS

- The dermatoscopic patterns of distal subungual onychomycosis help to determine which nails to sample for mycologic testing.
- For distal subungual onychomycosis specimens, the most specific dermatoscopic patterns were the "jagged edge with spikes" and "longitudinal striae."
- Subungual debris is the skin's inflammatory reaction pattern to the process of fungal invasion. One can best view this by positioning the dermatoscope at the distal edge of the nail plate.

REFERENCES

1. Ameen M, Lear JT, Madnan V, et al. British Association of Dermatologists' guidelines for the management of onychomycosis. Br J Dermatol 2014;171:937–58.
2. Piraccini BM, Balestri R, Starace M, et al. Nail digital dermoscopy (onychoscopy) in the diagnosis of onychomycosis. J Eur Acad Dermatol Venereol 2013;27(4): 509–13.
3. Kaynak E, Gotkay F, Gunes P, et al. The role of dermoscopy in the diagnosis of distal lateral subungual onychomycosis. Arch Dermatol Res 2018;310:57–69.
4. Yorulmaz A, Yalcin B. Dermoscopy as a first step in the diagnosis of onychomycosis. Adv Dermatol Allergol 2018;XXXV(3):251–8.
5. Piraccini BM, Alessandrini A, Bruni F, et al. Dermoscopy in the diagnosis of onychomycosis. In: Rigopoulos D, Elewski B, Richert B, editors. Onychomycosis: diagnosis and effective management. Hoboken (NJ): John Wiley & Sons; 2018. p. 66–73.
6. Bodman MA. Point-of-care diagnosis of onychomycosis by dermoscopy. J Am Podiatr Med Assoc 2017;107(5):413–8.

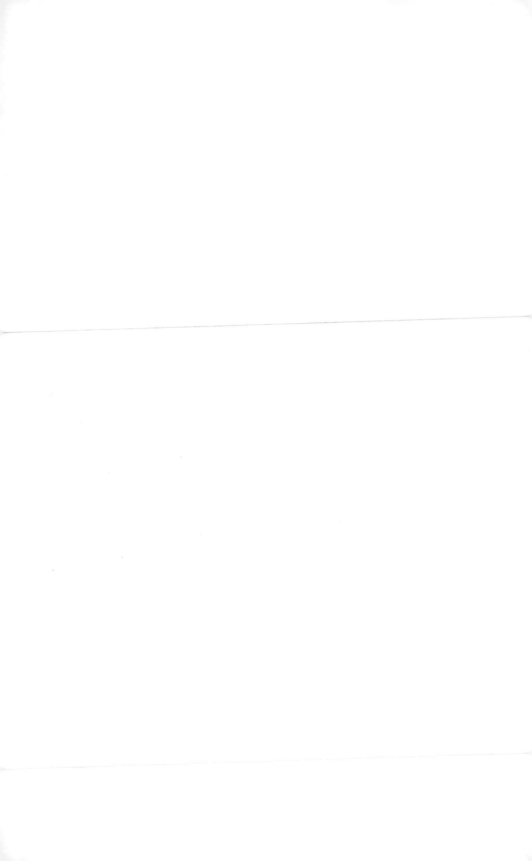

Plantar Verruca and Dermoscopy: An Update

Adam Bhatti, DPM, Saakshi Chowdhary, DPM,
Thomas Ferrise, DPM, Naga Govardhanam, DPM,
Alexandra Parish, DPM, Yaakov Tropper, DPM,
Tracey C. Vlahovic, DPM*

KEYWORDS

• Plantar warts • Plantar verrucae • Verruca • Dermoscopy • Dermatoscope

KEY POINTS

- The dermatoscope is a noninvasive tool used by dermatologists to inspect the surface features of the skin, including visualization of melanin located in the epidermis and dermis.
- The usage of the dermatoscope, in addition to the various algorithms and classifications, has made the process of narrowing down differential diagnoses much more accurate and precise not only for pigmented lesions but also for common lesions like warts.
- Once diagnosis and treatment of the wart have begun, the dermatoscope then allows the practitioner to follow the disappearance of the capillaries and honeycomb appearance and the restoration of the dermatoglyphics, which shows complete resolution of the wart and ultimately avoids premature cessation of treatment.

INTRODUCTION

The dermatoscope is a handheld tool that is used in dermatology to assess pigmented lesions. Traditionally, it is used to determine if a lesion is melanocytic or nonmelanocytic, and once this is established, recognizable patterns of the lesion are assessed to determine if a skin biopsy is warranted. Dermoscopy can be applied to skin issues like nail pathologic condition, skin rashes, and nonpigmented lesions. However, in both dermatology and podiatry, it is underused in the assessment of verrucae. The key to successful treatment of verrucae is first recognition of the lesion and finally its resolution after treatment. Traditionally, physicians have solely relied on more subjective features of verrucae for identification. The use of the dermatoscope has given physicians a more objective means of diagnosing and following the treatment course of warts. In accompaniment with clinical expertise, this pocket-sized device allows the physician to distinguish between verrucae, hyperkeratosis (ie, corns and calluses),

Conflict of interest: None of the authors have any financial interests to disclose for this article.
Temple University School of Podiatric Medicine, 148 North 8th Street, Philadelphia, PA 19107, USA
* Corresponding author.
E-mail address: traceyv@temple.edu

and other dermatologic pathologic conditions. Ultimately, the dermatoscope aids in documenting the progression and response to treatment to provide a well-tailored treatment plan for the patient.

WARTS

Warts, also known as verrucae, are one of the most frequent causes of dermatologic and podiatric visits. Most warts are caused by the human papilloma virus (HPV), and the subtypes responsible for most plantar warts are HPV strains 1, 2, 4, 27, and 57.[1] One of the key characteristics of warts is the "black dots" commonly seen within the superficial surface of the wart and which are used to help diagnose the infection. The black dots were historically thought to be thrombosed capillaries located in the dermal structures. However, recent studies have revealed that the black dots are not located in the dermal layer; rather, they are superficial hemorrhages located in the cornified layer of the skin.[2]

Plantar (or palmoplantar) warts are from the same HPV subtypes but often present with different characteristics (**Fig. 1**). The hallmark feature of palmoplantar warts is the firm papules located on the plantar surface of the foot, and these can coalesce into a plaque, which disrupts the normal dermatoglyphics of the skin.[3]

Other distinguishing characteristics that are seen in warts include a well-defined border that is elevated, rough, and flaky white in appearance. Most warts located on the plantar surface of the foot present with a hyperkeratotic covering, whereas common warts (located anywhere on the body besides the soles of the feet) more commonly are pink to flesh-colored in appearance.[4]

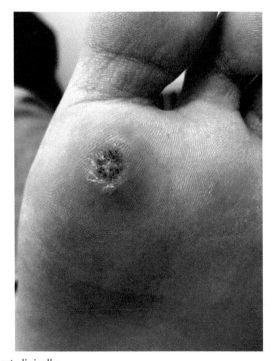

Fig. 1. Plantar wart clinically.

WARTS VERSUS CALLUSES

Calluses, or hyperkeratotic lesions, are the thickening of stratum corneum that appears on areas that are prone to excessive pressure, friction, or other constant irritation.[5] The stress on the skin will cause a proliferation and deposition of keratin in the epidermis in order to serve as a protective mechanism.[6] The presence of pain can be variable based on each individual patient. Calluses can appear hard, yellow, scaly, and thick.

Biomechanics and improper footwear are 2 common causes of callus formation.[5] Treatment of biomechanical issues with proper orthotics or padding will decrease the occurrence to a certain extent.[5] Traditionally, the lateral squeeze test method of the focal hyperkeratotic lesion has been a diagnostic tool widely used by physicians to distinguish between plantar warts and calluses.[7] The method involves applying direct perpendicular pressure first and eliciting a response from the patient followed by applying pressure to the left and right side of the lesion and eliciting a response from the patient.[7] Pressure with direct perpendicular pressure is indicative of a callus, whereas pressure on the sides of the lesion is traditionally indicative of a wart.[7] The lateral squeeze test is generally successful in distinguishing a wart versus a callus; however, there are times that the test elicits a positive response with both direct pressure and lateral pressure, which blurs the result.

Another distinguishing characteristic is the presence of "black dots" correlating with dilated capillaries in warts in comparison to calluses. Although these black dots are sometimes visible to the naked eye, they are not always present and could lead to an inaccurate diagnosis.[2] Skin lines or dermatoglyphics are traditionally seen running through a callus, whereas they are not present in a wart. Calluses are often seen in weight-bearing and traumatic areas on the foot.[8] These areas can include the first metatarsal head and fifth metatarsal base.[9] Warts, however, can be found in any area and do not correlate with increased weight-bearing pressure.

DERMOSCOPY

The dermatoscope is a noninvasive tool used by dermatologists to inspect the surface features of the skin, including visualization of melanin located in the epidermis and dermis.[10] The dermatoscope is a hand-held device composed of a magnifying lens and a light source. The lens of the dermatoscope commonly magnifies lesions 10- to 14-fold.[11] In addition to the lens and the light source, the lesion to be examined is covered in a fluid such as mineral oil, water, or alcohol (hand-sanitizer gel) in order to negate any reflection off the skin's surface, rendering the keratinized layer of the skin translucent and the melanocytic structures in the epidermal and dermal layers more visible11 (**Fig. 2**).

Dermoscopy, in conjunction with clinical diagnosis, helps physicians better visualize the features of a patient's skin in vivo that are not visible to the naked eye and improves diagnostic accuracy.[11] Traditionally, a dermatoscope is used in the diagnosis of pigmented skin lesions, particularly melanoma and seborrheic keratoses. Lallas and colleagues[12] noted that in addition to discerning areas of melanin deposition in the skin, dermatoscopes can also be used to examine "vascular alterations, color variegations, and follicle disturbances" in the epidermal and dermal layers.

To recognize the features of verrucae more objectively, it is imperative to also establish identification criteria upon which a physician can make a diagnosis. There are several different algorithms previously published regarding melanoma and pigmented lesion diagnosis using dermatoscopes. Pattern analysis is a widely accepted method used to differentiate between benign melanocytic lesions and melanomas. In addition, the ABCD rule (also known as the Stolz method) helps physicians determine the likelihood that a pigmented lesion is melanoma.[8] The Menzies algorithm attempts to

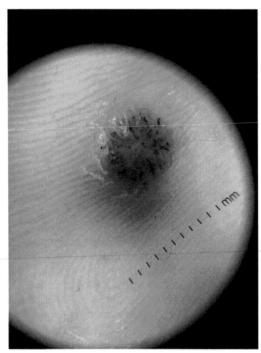

Fig. 2. The wart from **Fig. 1** via dermoscopy showing the capillary network and interruption of skin lines.

differentiate between benign and malignant lesions based on 2 negative (nonmelanotic) and 9 positive criteria (melanotic).[11] Diagnostic criterion such as these may be extrapolated and modified to formulate an objective, standardized set of rules for the diagnosis of verrucous skin lesions.

WART DERMOSCOPY

Following the establishment of the "2-step algorithm" for the classification of melanocytic lesions, the emergence of both polarized and nonpolarized light dermatoscopes revealed the need for further adjustments to ensure accurate diagnoses.[13] Thus, supplementary classifications were incorporated into the algorithm, allowing for thorough evaluation of amelanotic and hypomelanotic lesions.[13] Furthermore, deliberate examination of these lesions exposes an intricate network of capillaries, offering insight that these lesions contain structure and characteristic features.[13] The highest classification, level 7, is reserved for lesions demonstrating indiscernible features.[13]

As previously mentioned, cutaneous warts presenting on the plantar aspect of the foot traditionally exhibit comparable patterns of hyperkeratosis with those of calluses and corns.[14] Upon debridement of any of these lesions, the practitioner may need assistance in distinguishing a wart versus a callus, especially in the demographics of young children and the immunocompromised, which supports the need for a more streamlined diagnosis.[14] The dermatoscope allows for visualization of underlying capillaries associated with cutaneous warts that cannot always be seen by the unaided eye. Consequently, research concerning warts aims to describe the vascular observations elicited via the dermatoscope.[14] The introduction of the dermatoscope to evaluate warts exposes any network of capillaries that may exist.[15]

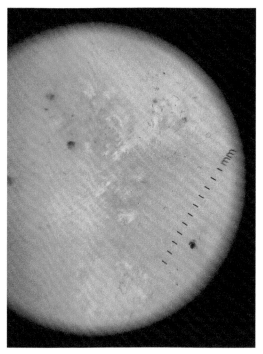

Fig. 3. Honeycomb appearance visible at 11 o'clock.

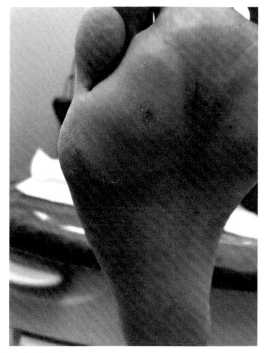

Fig. 4. Clinical lesion plantarly.

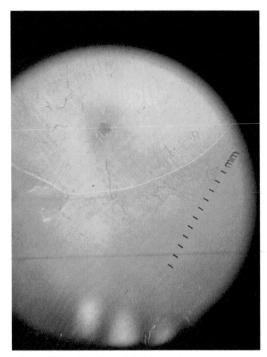

Fig. 5. Dermoscopic view of **Fig. 4** before debridement.

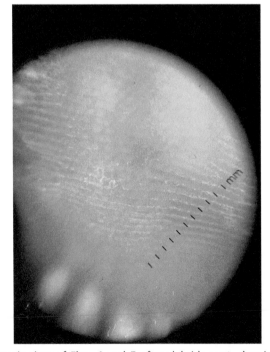

Fig. 6. Dermatoscopic view of **Figs. 4** and **5** after debridement, showing skin lines, thus showing the lesion is a focal hyperkeratotic lesion and not a wart.

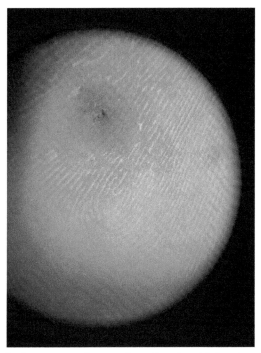

Fig. 7. After 1 month of treatment, the wart from **Figs. 1** and **2** showing skin lines traversing through most of the lesion with reduction of capillary network. The lesion is not fully resolved, but shows how much has changed in the space of a month.

In addition to visualizing capillary networks and interruption of dermatoglyphics, plantar warts have a characteristic "honeycomb"-like appearance on debridement[14] (**Figs. 3–6**). Once diagnosis and treatment of the wart have begun, the dermatoscope then allows the practitioner to follow the disappearance of the capillaries and honeycomb appearance and the restoration of the dermatoglyphics, which shows complete resolution of the wart and ultimately avoids premature cessation of treatment[14] (**Fig. 7**).

The usage of the dermatoscope, in addition to the various algorithms and classifications, has made the process of narrowing down differential diagnoses much more accurate and precise not only for pigmented lesions but also for common lesions like warts.[14]

SUMMARY

Although warts are a common occurrence in medicine, a foolproof method to diagnose and detect them is being formulated with the addition of dermoscopy. Physicians often rely on their personal preferences and choose from more subjective diagnostic methods, such as the lateral squeeze maneuver, punch biopsy, and even simple pattern recognition involving the assessment of color, border, and symmetry of the lesion to identify warts.[11] Although these methods are commonplace, they are more likely to be tainted with bias, relying on the physician's prior experiences and the patient's assessment of pain.

Using the dermatoscope as a standard and first-line tool of diagnosis can prove to be more promising in objectively and thoroughly assessing lesions as well as offering more effective treatment approaches. The tool, however, is only as competent as the physician using it. Therefore, along with standardizing the diagnostic approach, there remains a need to develop a set of mechanical guidelines for operating dermatoscopes in studying the nature of skin lesions like warts. Training future health care professionals in dermoscopy will bring the profession one step closer to a more unified approach to identifying and treating warts. This can lead to a better outcome in patient care and especially improve the mobility and quality of life in those suffering from plantar warts.

REFERENCES

1. Vlahovic T, Khan MT. The human papillomavirus and its role in plantar warts: a comprehensive review of diagnosis and management. Clin Podiatr Med Surg 2016;33:337–53.
2. Isabella Fried MR. Black dots in palmoplantar warts –challenging a concept: a histopathologic study. J Am Acad Dermatol 2018;79(2):380–2.
3. Yang FQ. Intralesional pingyangmycin treatment for resistant plantar warts. Dermatology 2010;220:110–3.
4. Hogendoorn GB. Morphological characteristics and human papillomavirus genotype predict the treatment response in cutaneous warts. Br J Dermatol 2018;178:253–60.
5. Simons SM, Kennedy R. Chapter 34 – foot injuries. In: Clinical Sports Medicine. ; 2007:473-489. Available at: https://www.sciencedirect.com/science/article/pii/B9781416024439500374.
6. Kirwan H, Pignataro R. Chapter 2 – the skin and wound healing. In: Pathology and Intervention in Musculoskeletal Rehabilitation. 2nd ed.; 2016:25-62. Available at: https://www.sciencedirect.com/science/article/pii/B9780323310727000026.
7. Zaiac MN, Mlacker S, Shah VV, et al. Clinical pearl: the squeeze maneuver. Cutis 2016;97(3):202–4. Available at: https://www.mdedge.com/cutis/article/107174/aesthetic-dermatology/clinical-pearl-squeeze-maneuver.
8. Other algorithms for melanocytic lesions CME. DermNet New Zealand website. Available at: https://www.dermnetnz.org/cme/dermoscopy-course/other-algorithms-for-melanocytic-lesions/. Accessed April 10, 2018.
9. Amemiya A, Okonogi R, Yamakawa H, et al. The external force associated with callus formation under the first metatarsal head is reduced by wearing rocker sole shoes. 2017 39th Annual International Conference of the IEEE Engineering in Medicine and Biology Society (EMBC). 2017. https://doi.org/10.1109/embc.2017.8037853.
10. Chiṭu V, Zurac S, Cipi AE. Dermatoscopy of verrucous pigmented lesions is essential for choosing the appropriate treatment. Rom J Intern Med 2015;53(4). https://doi.org/10.1515/rjim-2015-0047.
11. Argenziano G, Soyer HP. Dermoscopy of pigmented skin lesions – a valuable tool for early. Lancet Oncol 2001;2(7):443–9. https://doi.org/10.1016/s1470-2045(00)00422-8.
12. Lallas A, Zalaudek I, Argenziano G, et al. Dermoscopy in general dermatology. Dermatol Clin 2013;31(4):679–94.
13. Marghoob AA, Braun R. Proposal for a revised 2-step algorithm for the classification of lesions of the skin using dermoscopy. Arch Dermatol 2010;146(4):426–8.
14. Bae J, Kang H, Kim H, et al. Differential diagnosis of plantar wart from corn, callus and healed wart with the aid of dermoscopy. Br J Dermatol 2009;160(1):220–2.
15. Lee D-Y, Park J-H, Lee J-H, et al. The use of dermoscopy for the diagnosis of plantar wart. J Eur Acad Dermatol Venereol 2009;23(6):726–7.

Disappearing Nail Bed
Review of Etiology, Grading System, and Treatment Options

Flavia Filisio, DPM, Shelby Busch, DPM,
Delaney J.H. Wickramage, DPM, Russell Hill, DPM,
Sushila Kabadi, DPM, Carolina Lordelo Van Pelt, DPM,
Tracey C. Vlahovic, DPM*

KEYWORDS

- Disappearing nail bed • Onycholysis • Onychomycosis • Toenail

KEY POINTS

- Disappearing nail bed occurs after long standing onycholysis.
- DNB can occur in the fingernails and toenails.
- Patients often complain of pain at the distal border of the nail and that the nail won't grow forward.

INTRODUCTION

Disappearing nail bed (DNB) is the phenomenon of nail bed epithelialization following prolonged onycholysis, or separation of the nail plate from the nail bed (**Fig. 1**). It presents clinically as a shortened or narrowed nail bed.[1] In addition to causing cosmetic concern for patients, DNB is also associated with the development of onychomycosis, distal paronychia, and other pathologic conditions.

A firm understanding of the nail anatomy is necessary in order to distinguish between different nail pathologic conditions and appropriate treatment methods. The nail unit consists of the nail plate, nail bed, surrounding soft tissue folds, and neurovasculature.[2] The nail plate is a laminated keratinized structure that overlies the nail bed and nail matrix. A normal nail bed does not have a granular layer. The nail plate can often become separated from the nail bed. This separation is termed onycholysis and has many possible causes: infection, exposure to contact irritants, systemic disease, or the use of certain drugs and medications.[3] When distal onycholysis occurs

Conflict of Interest: None of the authors have any financial interests to disclose for this article.
Temple University School of Podiatric Medicine, 148 North 8th Street, Philadelphia, PA 19107, USA
* Corresponding author.
E-mail address: traceyv@temple.edu

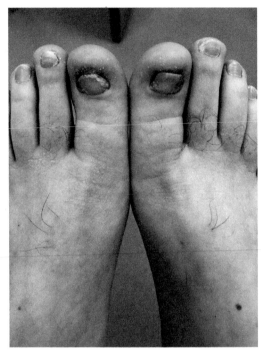

Fig. 1. Bilateral presentation of DNB on both halluces.

and is not treated promptly, the nail bed can epithelialize and develop dermato-glyphics, or finger/toe prints. This process was first described in 2005 by Daniel and colleagues[3] and was termed DNB.

Although there is still relatively little literature regarding DNB, there have been several studies examining the cause and treatment of onycholysis that have implications for DNB. This review examines the cause, classification system, and possible treatment methods that have been described for onycholysis and DNB.

CAUSE

Onycholysis can be diagnosed clinically with relative ease based on the opaque, white appearance of the portion of the nail plate, which has separated from the underlying nail bed. Although onycholysis is a commonly seen pathologic condition, the exact incidence of both onycholysis and DNB is unknown. The condition can affect both the fingernails and the toenails. Onycholysis of the fingernails is more commonly seen in women and is most often caused by trauma.[4] This trauma can be the result of fingernail care and/or manicures, occupational activities, or onychotillomania (a nervous tic). The condition is often further exacerbated by patient attempts at self-guided treatment using topical products or by cutting the separated portion of the nail plate. Numerous additional causes have been attributed to the development of onycholysis of the fingernails, including the use of certain drugs (such as tetracyclines, paclitaxel, psoralens, aminolevulinic acid, aripiprazole, 5-fluorouracil, griseofulvin, oral contraceptives), photodermatitis, allergic contact dermatitis precipitated by exposure to various chemicals, and irritant contact dermatitis from prolonged immersion of nails in water. In addition, onycholysis has been noted to occur secondary to dermatologic conditions, such as psoriasis and lichen planus.[4] For onycholysis resulting from any of the above listed conditions, treatment of the primary condition and/or removal of the causative drug or irritant is the first step in correcting the condition. For simple onycholysis not produced by a known disease, keeping nails short and avoiding irritating stimuli are recommended.[5] In addition, ensuring thorough drying of hands to prevent moisture from being trapped under the nail can prevent an overgrowth of microbial flora. A moist warm environment under the nail bed can allow the entry and colonization of organisms such as *Candida albicans* or *Pseudomonas*.[4]

Although toenail onycholysis can also be associated with trauma to the nail unit, the causes of trauma to the nails of the foot are unique and separate from those affecting the fingernails. Tight, closed shoes exerting pressure on the toes as result of uneven flat feet is 1 possible cause of onycholysis of the toenails. This process has been described as asymmetric gait nail unit syndrome.[4] In addition to trauma, other possible causes include onychogryphosis, biomechanics (eg, hallux extensus) (**Fig. 2**), nail surgery (iatrogenic trauma), and onychomycosis (Tracey C. Vlahovic, DPM, personal communication, 2017). The opening beneath the nail plate created by onycholysis can provide an opening for opportunistic infection by dermatophytes, most commonly *Trichophyton rubrum*, resulting in onychomycosis. Onychomycosis in turn can result in the development or worsening of onycholysis of the toenails (**Fig. 3**).

Without proper treatment and resolution, onycholysis can ultimately result in DNB syndrome. In a 2016 study of 540 patients seen in a dermatology clinic in Mississippi, 13.15% (71 out of 540) presented with DNB of 1 or more nails.[1] DNB in this study was described as a nail that is 20% shorter or narrower than the same nail of the opposite hand or foot.[1] Of those with DNB, 63.34% were men and 46.36% were women. Although differences in gender were not shown to be statistically significant, a

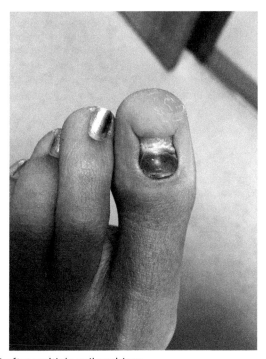

Fig. 2. Hallux DNB after multiple nail avulsions.

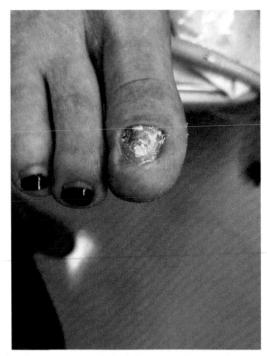

Fig. 3. DNB following long-term onycholysis from onychomycosis.

statistically significant correlation was found between age and DNB, with 69.25 years old being the average age of patients presenting with the condition. Of the 11 patients with DNB of 1 or more fingernails, the majority reported a history of onychophagia (biting of the nails). Trauma and onychotillomania were also commonly reported in these patients' histories. Onychomycosis was found in approximately one-third of patients (22 out of 60) presenting with DNB of 1 or more toenails. Also commonly reported in patients with DNB of the toes was a history of trauma, previous surgery, or onychogryphosis (**Fig. 4**).

GRADING SYSTEM

Although it has been established that untreated or longstanding onycholysis is associated with the development of DNB, the time needed for this progression to occur has not been studied. However, the stages have been observed, and the advancement of initial onycholysis to DNB has been documented into a grading system.[6]

The grading system is as follows:

- Stage I: early, initial separation of 1 to 2 mm of the distal nail plate from the hyponychium
- Stage II: separation of the distal one-third of the nail plate
- Stage III: separation of one-third to two-thirds of the nail plate
- Stage IV: onycholysis extending from the proximal nail fold to the distal end of the nail
- Stage V: development of DNB, including cornification of a portion of the nail bed or hyponychium, and development of dermatoglyphics like those seen on the tip of the digit

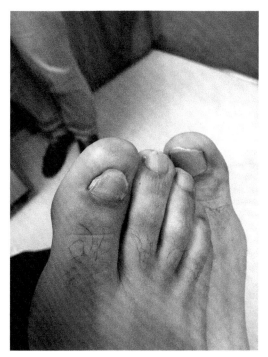

Fig. 4. Patients often complain of pain at the distal border of the nail plate where it impinges on the skin.

DNB and onycholysis are difficult to treat if not correctly diagnosed in a timely manner. A proper history along with clinical findings of the nail and surrounding tissues is essential for correct management and treatment. Therefore, a grading system based on clinical findings, such as the one described above, helps the physician to evaluate the progression of the patient's condition and prescribe the correct treatment options for their specific stage of onycholysis.

TREATMENT METHODS

In addition to many conservative options, several surgical treatments have been described for the management of DNB. The conservative options include taping of the distal skin of the digit using medical grade retention tape, wearing shoes with a wide toe box in order to accommodate the deformity and prevent further trauma, and camouflaging with a cosmetic nail resin (Keryflex) for cosmetic purposes (Tracey C. Vlahovic, DPM, personal communication). (**Fig. 5**). As DNB progresses, the distal pulp of the toe enlarges and deforms. This enlargement and deformity create a physical barrier when the nail grows forward and predisposes the digit to the development of a distal paronychia. One conservative method that has been attempted is taping of the skin distal to the nail plate in order to elongate the skin away from the plate and reduce the size of the distal pulp (Tracey C. Vlahovic, DPM, personal communication).

If conservative methods fail or prove insufficient, several surgical treatment options have been described. These methods include serial excisions, the application of gingival grafts or artificial dermis to attempt to recreate the nail bed, or the excision of a distal wedge of the skin in order to advance skin distally and prevent distal ingrowth of toenails (Tracey C. Vlahovic, DPM, personal communication).

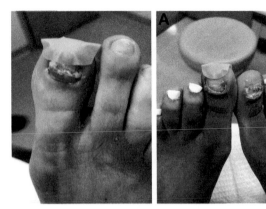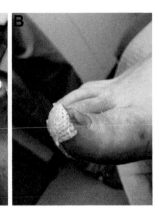

Fig. 5. Taping method for DNB.

If there is still a portion of the nail bed exhibiting growth in the region of the lunula, serial excisions can be performed in order to elongate the nail. This technique was used in 11 partially destroyed nail beds between 1990 and 1994, 6 of which were due to mycosis and 5 of which were due to trauma.[7] A crescent-shaped excision 5 mm at its greatest width, extending from 1 lateral nail fold to the other and down to the periosteum, can be performed in order to remove scarred nail tissue directly adjacent to the healthy nail. After regeneration of the new nail bed and nail plate over 2 to 3 months, a second excision of the remaining distal scar tissue is performed. This study reported no failures or complications, and normal nail growth was achieved in all 11 patients. The technique aims to take advantage of the unidirectional growth vectors of the proximal nail bed. This type of growth allows healthy nail bed to replace the defect created by excision of the scarred nail bed faster than the multidirectional growth of the distal granulation tissue.

The use of a hard palate graft is another surgical option that has shown potential to be effective in the treatment of nail bed defects. In a longitudinal study in 2006, 7 nails with nail dystrophy or permanent onycholysis were treated using a hard palate mucosal graft in order to remove the scarred portion of the nail bed and induce adherence of the nail plate to the nail bed.[8] An otolaryngologist harvested the hard palate mucosal graft. The affected portion of the nail bed was then resected, and the defect was covered by an equivalently sized graft. It was sutured using 7-0 Vicryl suture. Six fingernails and 1 toenail were repaired, and follow-up was done at 7 days, 2 weeks, and every month until the nail had grown out completely. At follow-up, acceptable nail growth and improved adherence were noted. All patients were pleased with the results. This technique has been attempted elsewhere and reported to achieve satisfactory results.[5]

Another technique that has been attempted is the use of artificial dermis. This method was explored in a retrospective study of 22 patients between 2004 and 2009 with injuries to the proximal half of the nail bed.[9] The injuries treated were classified into 3 types. Type 1, of which 8 were included in the study, involved relatively distal defects that were localized to the nail bed. The treatment and results of this type are most applicable to the discussion of treatments for DNB. In these cases, scarred nail bed was excised, and artificial dermis was applied to the defect and fixed using 5-0 nylon suture.[9] In all cases, it was reported that the nail was regenerated almost completely, and patients were satisfied with the results. No difference in clinical outcomes was seen between the 2 types of artificial dermis used.

SUMMARY

Although DNB is likely a common phenomenon, relatively little research has been dedicated to the topic since it was first described in 2005 by Daniel and colleagues Although some of the existing literature regarding cause, classification system, and treatment options was discussed above, there remains the potential for further exploration of how the condition is initiated, progresses, and is best managed.

A lack of data exists regarding the incidence of DNB in the population as well as how long the progression from onycholysis to DNB takes. Additional studies are also necessary to better understand the factors associated with the development of DNB and what causes onycholysis to progress to this stage in certain patients. In addition, studies of current treatment options are somewhat limited in their impact by small sample sizes and measures of outcomes that are qualitative (based on patient satisfaction or general nail appearance) rather than quantitative. Further research comparing different treatment modalities in terms of outcome, recovery time, and complication rates could be useful to clinicians in making treatment decisions to best address their patients' needs.

CLINICS CARE POINTS

- Rule out if there is a subungual exostosis present.
- Set realistic expectations with the patient regarding growth of nail and appearance.
- Discuss the array of conservative and surgical options available with the patient.

REFERENCES

1. Daniel R, Meir B, Avner S. An update on the disappearing nail bed. Skin Appendage Disord 2017;3(1):15–7.
2. de Berker D. Nail anatomy. Clin Dermatol 2013;31(5):509–15.
3. Daniel R, Tosti A, Iorizzo M, et al. The disappearing nail bed: a possible outcome of onycholysis. Cutis 2005;76:325–7.
4. Zaias N, Escovar S, Zaiac M. Finger and toenail onycholysis. J Eur Acad Dermatol Venereol 2015;29(5):848–53.
5. Dominguez-Cherit J, Daniel CR. Simple onycholysis: an attempt at surgical intervention. J Dermatol Surg 2010;36:1791–3.
6. Daniel R, Iorizzo M, Piraccini B, et al. Grading simple chronic paronychia and onycholysis. Int J Dermatol 2006;45:1447–8.
7. Lemperle G, Schwarz M, Lemperle S. Nail regeneration by elongation of the partially destroyed nail bed. Plast Reconstr Surg 2003;111(1):167072, discussion 173.
8. Fernandez-Mejia S, Dominguez-Cherit J, Pichardo-Velazques P, et al. Treatment of nail bed defects with hard palate mucosal grafts. J Cutan Med Surg 2006;10(2): 69–72.
9. Sugamata A. Regeneration of nails with artificial dermis. J Plast Surg Hand Surg 2012;46(3–4):191–4.

Biofilms and the Nail Unit

Corinna Castillo, DPM, Michael F. Masi, DPM, Austin Mishko, DPM,
Alex Sheltzer, DPM, Alex Speer, DPM, Heather Tran, DPM, Tracey C. Vlahovic, DPM*

KEYWORDS

- Biofilms • Bacterial biofilm • Fungal biofilm • Biofilm therapies • Onychomycosis
- Nails • *Candida albicans*

KEY POINTS

- Biofilms produce an extracellular matrix that serves as protection against host immunologic defenses.
- Because biofilms are often formed by multiple organisms, such as fungal and bacterial, and because drugs are less effective at penetrating the biofilm structure.
- There are no standardized treatments specifically for onychomycosis with biofilm formation, as more research is needed.

INTRODUCTION

The role of biofilms in disease pathogenesis remains a key component in better understanding microbial resistance to drug treatment. Biofilms are characterized as a collection of surface-adherent microorganisms enclosed by an extracellular, polymeric matrix.[1] Typical areas of biofilm formation include living tissue, fragments of dead tissue, and indwelling medical devices, such as catheters or prosthetic implants.[1,2] Although biofilms traditionally pertain to bacterial microorganisms, recent studies indicate that fungi, similar to their bacterial counterparts, also form biofilms alternating between planktonic and multicellular communities.[3] In pathogenic fungi such as *Candida albicans*, biofilm formation involves adherence to an abiotic or mucosal surface, yeast cell proliferation, and initiation of hyphal formation,[4] resulting in a dense network of yeasts, hyphae, and pseudohyphae.[5] Several genes encoding transcription factors, cell-wall biogenesis proteins, adherence proteins, and metabolic genes, including those for amino acid synthesis, remain conserved biofilm regulators across various fungal species.[4] The unique structure and intrinsic bioregulation of fungal biofilms are thought to enhance fungal adherence to mammalian cells and allow for infection to persist.[2,3]

Conflict of interest: None of the authors have any financial interests to disclose for this article.
Temple University School of Podiatric Medicine, 148 North 8th Street, Philadelphia, PA 19107, USA
* Corresponding author.
E-mail address: traceyv@temple.edu

Biofilm Pathogenesis

Bacterial and fungal biofilms possess characteristics that allow for a unique pathogenesis, which are difficult for immune mechanisms to handle. Once adhered to a foreign substance, biofilms produce an extracellular matrix that serves as protection against host immunologic defenses, such as phagocytosis and opsonization.[3] Studies have shown that biofilms consisting of staphylococcal species are less effective in generating the protective extracellular matrix and less efficient in evading the host's immune mechanisms.[3] Thus, virulence of biofilms may potentially depend on extracellular matrix formation and quality.

Genetic and environmental factors also influence the ability of certain species to form biofilms. For example, attachment to polystyrene by *Saccharomyces cerevisiae* is dependent on the FLO11 gene, which encodes fungal cell surface glycoproteins.[2] In addition, biofilm formation was absent when *S cerevisiae* was placed in an environment lacking glucose.[2] *C albicans* possesses an ortholog of the FLO11 gene that may enhance its virulence in mammalian cells, such as nail units.[2]

Candida species are among the most common causes of fungal biofilm infections.[6] Factors conferring resistance to drug treatment and persistence of infection include biofilm architectural complexity, metabolic heterogeneity, and upregulation of multidrug-resistant efflux pumps.[4] Fungal biofilms have increasingly significant clinical implications because of the opportunistic nature of their pathogenicity and their increasing resistance to antifungal therapies.[5,6]

ONYCHOMYCOSIS

Onychomycosis is an infection of the nail often caused by fungal species and accounts for roughly 50% of all nail diseases universally.[7–9] Although *Trichophyton rubrum* is often the offending organism, onychomycosis can be caused by various fungal pathogens, including other dermatophytes, nondermatophyte molds, or yeasts such as *Candida* species.[7,8] *C albicans* is among the most common etiologic agents in onychomycosis with *Candida* species found in approximately 75% of all nail infections.[7]

Epidemiology

Individuals susceptible to fungal biofilm infections primarily are often immunocompromised. Immunocompromised individuals include patients with HIV/AIDS, cancer, peripheral vascular disease, diabetes mellitus; those taking immunosuppressive drug treatment; the elderly; smokers; and hospitalized patients who develop nosocomial infections.[3,7,10]

Other important factors that may increase the risk of nail biofilm formation include physical damage and insult to the nail and concurrent infection with other microorganisms. Exposure to *C albicans* during cuticle removal with improperly sterilized equipment during a manicure also presents a risk.[7] Other physical factors include nail trauma, dryness of nail from normal aging, nail overhydration, removal of protective lipids on the nail from soaking, and any other interference of a normal nail barrier.[11] Concurrent tinea pedis infection may infect the nail by producing mycotoxins that damage the nail externally, thus making biofilm formation more likely.[7,11]

Diagnosis

Patient evaluation

A complete history and physical examination are pertinent when evaluating a patient for onychomycosis.[12] It is important to note how long the patient has been experiencing symptoms, such as pain or discomfort, as well as his/her medical history. Regarding nail disease, 50% is caused by onychomycosis, whereas the other half is caused by conditions that mimic onychomycosis.[12] Differential diagnoses may include other skin conditions, such as psoriasis and eczema, which mimic mycotic nails in their clinical presentations.[12,13] Gait biomechanics should also be assessed before suspecting onychomycosis. Repeated microtrauma from poor biomechanics can cause the appearance of the nails to look dystrophic and mycotic,[12] thus making thorough evaluation of the nails essential in ruling out other suspected pathologic conditions.

Nail fungal culture

To confirm the presence of onychomycosis, primary diagnostic methods include KOH tests, PAS stains, or fungal cultures of biopsy samples.[12] The biopsy process involves cleaning the affected area with 70% isopropyl alcohol and obtaining samples of infected nail and subungual debris[13] via use of punch biopsy, excisional biopsy, or nail avulsion techniques. Microscopy and KOH staining confirm the presence of infection but use of PAS staining and culture is required to identify the infecting organism. Once the organism has been identified, a targeted treatment regimen can be implemented, or another nail disorder can be considered.[13]

Treatment

Although there are no standardized treatments specifically for onychomycosis with biofilm formation, Miltefosine has been shown to have the most promise in laboratory studies. It is able to both prevent formation of and lessen preexisting *C albicans* and *Fusarium oxysporum* biofilm infections on human fingernail fragments.[7] Miltefosine has also been shown to be active against *T rubrum* and *Trichophyton mentagrophytes* while they are in planktonic form.[7] Miltefosine side effects are mostly related to the gastrointestinal tract, but are still less severe than those of amphotericin B. Its mechanism of action against fungal species is proposed to be from activation of the MCA1 (present in *C albicans*) and therefore causing a fungal cell death that resembles apoptosis.[7]

Lasers have also had some success in vitro against fungal species like *C albicans* and *F oxysporum.* Both 1064-nm Nd:YAG and 420-nm intense pulsed light followed by Nd:YAG were shown to be successful in treating human fingernail fragments in vitro. Although still under investigation, the mechanism of action for laser therapy is proposed to involve direct fungicidal effect via apoptosis owing to heat.[8]

Recent areas of research point toward essential oils as an attractive target for antibacterial biofilm therapy.[14] Plant-based essential oils, like cassia, Peru balsam, and red thyme, were shown in vitro to effectively treat the bacterial components of biofilms. In treating biofilms caused by *Pseudomonas aeruginosa* and *Staphylococcus aureus*, these plant-based oils eradicated bacteria within the biofilm at a higher efficiency than several antibiotics, including gentamicin, colistin, ofloxacin, and ampicillin. Although these initial studies have only examined bacterial biofilms, use of essential oils in biofilm treatment may apply similarly to fungal species as well.[14]

Resistance

Because biofilms are often formed by multiple organisms, such as fungal and bacterial, and because drugs are less effective at penetrating the biofilm structure, a nail biofilm, in theory, can be very difficult to treat.[11] Studies suggest that "azole" antifungal agents like fluconazole are not effective in treating *C albicans*–infected nails if a biofilm is present.[7] It has also been shown that itraconazole, voriconazole, and terbinafine are not effective in treating *F oxysporum* in the presence of a biofilm.[7] Onychomycosis in patients with diabetes presents resistance issues of its own and is amplified when biofilm formation is present. In one case, a patient died of fusarium after a combination of amphotericin B and voriconazole was unable to treat it.[8]

SUMMARY

The lack of standardized treatment and lack of intensive research for fungal biofilms and growing resistance to antifungal therapy necessitate further investigation into developing more effective antibiofilm therapies.[15]

With an increased understanding of fungal biofilms and their pathogenicity, additional therapies can be developed to address the present issue of antimicrobial resistance and provide improved outcomes in patients suffering from persistent onychomycosis infection.

CLINICS CARE POINTS

- Studies suggest that "azole" antifungal agents like fluconazole are not effective in treating C albicans–infected nails if a biofilm is present.
- Recent areas of research point toward essential oils as an attractive target for antibacterial biofilm therapy.
- The lack of standardized treatment and lack of intensive research for fungal biofilms and growing resistance to antifungal therapy necessitate further investigation into developing more effective therapies.

REFERENCES

1. Donlan RM. Biofilms: microbial life on surfaces. Emerg Infect Dis 2002;8(9): 881–90.
2. Reynolds TB, Fink GR. Bakers' yeast, a model for fungal biofilm formation. Science 2001;291(5505):878. Available at: http://link.galegroup.com.libproxy.temple.edu/apps/doc/A70696192/BIC?u=temple_main&sid=BIC&xid=02d52823.
3. Gupta AK, Daigle D, Carviel JL. The role of biofilms in onychomycosis. J Am Acad Dermatol 2016;74(6):1241–6.
4. Fanning S, Mitchell AP. Fungal biofilms. PLoS Pathog 2012;8(4):e1002585.
5. Jabra-Rizk MA, Falkler WA, Meiller TF. Fungal biofilms and drug resistance. Emerg Infect Dis 2004;10(1):14–9.
6. Ramage G, Mowat E, Jones B, et al. Our current understanding of fungal biofilms. Crit Rev Microbiol 2009;35(4):340–55.
7. Vila TV, Rozental S, Quintanilha NS. Miltefosine is effective against Candida albicans and Fusarium oxysporum nail biofilms in vitro. J Med Microbiol 2015;64(11): 1436–49.
8. Vila TV, Rozental S, De Sá Guimarães CM. A new model of in vitro fungal biofilms formed on human nail fragments allows reliable testing of laser and light therapies against onychomycosis. Lasers Med Sci 2014;30(3):1031–9.
9. Ghannoum MA, Hajjeh RA, Scher R, et al. A large-scale North American study of fungal isolates from nails: the frequency of onychomycosis, fungal distribution, and antifungal susceptibility patterns. J Am Acad Dermatol 2000;43:641–8.
10. Kaur R, Goyal R, Dhakad MS, et al. Epidemiology and virulence determinants including biofilm profile of Candida infections in an ICU in a tertiary hospital in India. J Mycol 2014;2014:1–8.
11. Burkhart CN, Burkhart CG, Gupta AK. Dermatophytoma: recalcitrance to treatment because of existence of fungal biofilm. J Am Acad Dermatol 2002;47(4): 629–31.

12. Vlahovic TC, July. Onychomycosis: evaluation, treatment options, managing recurrence, and patient outcomes. Clin Podiatric Med Surg 2016;33(3):305–18.
13. Westerberg DP, Voyack MJ. Onychomycosis: current trends in diagnosis and treatment. Am Fam Physician 2013;88(11):762–70.
14. Kavanaugh NL, Ribbeck K. Selected antimicrobial essential oils eradicate Pseudomonas spp. and Staphylococcus aureus biofilms. Appl Environ Microbiol 2012; 78(11):4057–61.
15. Arnaouteli S, Ferreira AS, Schoer M, et al. Bifunctionality of a biofilm matrix protein controlled by redox state 2017. Available at: http://www.pnas.org/content/early/2017/07/10/1707687114.

The Penetrance of Topical Nail Therapy
Limitations and Current Enhancements

Kari Phan, DPM, Kushkaran Kaur, DPM, Kayla Wright, DPM,
Son Tran, DPM, Benton Stewart, DPM, Michael Brown, DPM,
Tracey C. Vlahovic, DPM*

KEYWORDS

- Onychomycosis • Toenail • Keratin binding • Hydrophilic • Lipophilic • Antifungal

KEY POINTS

- Pharmaceuticals with a higher molecular weight and decreased polarity do not penetrate through the nail as well as substances with a lower molecular weight and increased polarity.
- Topical treatments for nail diseases must be specially formulated because of the thick nail plate barrier and the possible drug-binding affinity for keratin.
- Antifungal medications like efinaconazole and tavaborole have shown favorable use because of their low molecular weight and hydrophilicity, which leads to better transit across the nail plate.

INTRODUCTION

Nails are an epidermal derivative that serve as a protective barrier for the distal phalanges of toes and fingers.[1] Although they only make up a small portion of the human body, nail diseases comprise approximately 10% of all dermatologic pathologic conditions. In the lower extremities, the 2 most common disorders that affect toenails are onychomycosis and psoriasis.[2] Onychomycosis is a fungal infection that accounts for 50% of all nail diseases, with *Trichophyton rubrum* and *Trichophyton mentagrophytes* being the most common pathogens.[3,4] Patients may present with dystrophic nails, yellow-brown discoloration of the nail plate, and/or onycholysis. Although symptoms are non-life-threatening, affected patients are often embarrassed in both personal and work environments, leading to reduced self-confidence and an increased frequency of sick leave.[5,6]

Conflict of Interest: None of the authors have any financial interests to disclose for this article.
Temple University School of Podiatric Medicine, 148 North 8th Street, Philadelphia, PA 19107, USA
* Corresponding author.
E-mail address: traceyv@temple.edu

In contrast, psoriasis is a chronic inflammatory disease that affects all organs with the most apparent presentation on the skin and nails.[7] About 90% of patients with psoriasis are estimated to present with nail symptoms in their lifetime. Individuals with nail psoriasis complain of pain and suffer from social embarrassment, with 58% of patients reporting job interference because of the disease.[8] Furthermore, the rate of nail growth is increased in the presence of psoriasis.[9] Nail psoriasis and onychomycosis present with similar physical symptoms. However, psoriasis-affected nails additionally show signs of pitting, which is the characteristic loss of superficial nail matrix owing to the bursts of punctate foci.[10]

Treatments of both nail psoriasis and onychomycosis have focused on noninvasive therapies, such as topical solutions and lacquer, to avoid adverse effects that accompany systemic therapies. However, penetration of the nail plate has long been considered a barrier for effective topical therapy.[9] This review discusses the physiology of the nail and assesses how nail penetration can be improved with different vehicles of delivery.

BARRIERS TO NAIL PENETRATION

There are many factors that affect the penetration of topical medications across the nail, including molecular weight, polarity, and lipid content. Pharmaceuticals with a higher molecular weight and decreased polarity do not penetrate through the nail as well as substances with a lower molecular weight and increased polarity.[9,11] Furthermore, onychomycosis causes a change in the nail plate that influences the types of molecules that can penetrate through. In a study exploring how fungal infection influences drug penetration through diseased nail plates, it was observed that onychomycosis causes a tortuous, porous network in the nail. This allows small polar hydrophilic molecules, such as caffeine, to permeate through the diseased nail plates better and with a shorter lag time than through healthy nails. In contrast, no change was observed with lipophilic drugs, terbinafine and amorolfine, in their ability to penetrate the diseased nail versus the healthy nail. This supports the hypothesis that lipophilic drugs use keratin binding as a mode of transport through the nail plate, whereas small hydrophilic molecules can take advantage of the changed diseased nail structure.[12] Therefore, it is suggested that when treating a patient's nail, drug delivery can be enhanced with the use of low-molecular-weight and hydrophilic drug compounds for a more beneficial outcome.

Diseases such as onychomycosis and psoriasis alter the barrier functionality of the nail, which affects the efficacy of drug penetrance. These diseases also affect the skin, even though the skin has a markedly different biological structure than nails. Under the stress of diseases such as onychomycosis or psoriasis, the nail forms a stratum granulosum layer to prevent water loss through the secretion of lipids that is absent in healthy nails. Measurement of transonychial water loss (TOWL) can be performed to observe this alteration in barrier function and was significantly lower in nails affected by atopic eczema, psoriasis, and onychomycosis, compared with healthy nails.[13] Transepidermal water loss was significantly higher in skin affected by these same diseases, suggesting a decrease in barrier function in the diseased skin.[13] Because of dramatically different changes in skin compared with nail structure under disease stages, substances that enhance permeability through the skin do not act similarly on the nail. In an experiment showing that solvents that enhance permeability through the stratum corneum do not have the same effect on the nail plate, dimethyl sulfoxide, a solvent that increases the rate of drug diffusion through skin, was tested on nails. The difference in permeability can be attributed to the nail's lower lipid content than that of the skin.[14] It can also be postulated that the thickness, along with the higher cysteine and sulfur contents of the nail, compared with the stratum corneum of the skin, plays a role in the decreased concentration of topical drugs in the lower layers of the nail plate. It has been found that the concentration of topical therapies may decrease by 1000-fold from the top of the nail to the bottom.[15] It can be concluded that the nail's barrier structure is significantly different from that of the skin under the stress of disease processes, and different modes of penetration should be considered for nails than those used for skin.

Because drugs become inactive when bound to keratin, it has also been shown that drug penetration through the nail is reduced based on the ability of the drug to bind to keratin.[12,16] Furthermore, lipophilic drugs that bind to keratin and use it to travel exhibit decreased penetration through the nail.[12] Because of the decreased penetration through nails that are highly keratinized, it is recommended that the application of topical treatments should be started early in the disease progression. In addition, topical medications can be applied specifically onto the affected parts of the nail. Topical treatments have many benefits compared with oral medications, such as reducing the patient's risk of systemic side effects and drug-drug interactions.[9] Therefore, it is beneficial to treat any nail condition early in the disease process with topical drugs that do not bind keratin or do not have a high affinity to keratin.

METHODS TO ENHANCE NAIL PENETRATION: MECHANICAL, PHYSICAL, AND CHEMICAL
Mechanical

The nail plate is made of approximately 80 to 90 layers of keratin, making it difficult for topicals to penetrate the nail compared with skin.[17] Thickness of the dorsal layer of the nail makes penetration of topicals difficult; therefore, the nail is often filed down with a Dremel device or a nail file before application of drug compounds. In vitro this doubles the permeability coefficient of 5-fluorouracil and flurbiprofen through the nail plate.[18] In the presence of a fungal infection, abrasion of the nail plate can reduce the critical fungal mass, resulting in increased topical penetrance.[19] Hence, for a quality treatment of the dystrophic fungal nail, it is a beneficial practice to file the dorsum of the nail and thereby increase the drug permeability.

Physical

Physical enhancements may include iontophoresis, acid etching, carbon dioxide laser, microporation, microneedle, microsurgical laser, and/or low-frequency ultrasound. The efficacy of iontophoresis in enhancing the transport of small, charged molecules across the nail plate was demonstrated in an experiment observing in vivo iontophoresis. Researchers chose to use whole nails because nail plate thickness increases distal to proximal, and therefore, hydration at the free edge is different from the attached nail plate. Compared with the control group, iontophoresis significantly increased the amount of transungual transport of Na^+ and Cl^-. This shows the potential for enhancing drug delivery of small, charged molecules with iontophoresis. Researchers observed that iontophoresis is well tolerated by patients and does not alter TOWL.[20] In addition, a similar study showed that iontophoresis can allow Na^+ and Li^{2+} ions to diffusely penetrate the nail plate and permeate through the skin.[21] Therefore, iontophoresis is a reasonable and safe method of enhancing drug delivery across the nail plate.

In a study by Vanstone and colleagues,[22] it was shown that laser poration with a 1064-nm Fianium laser may also enhance drug delivery to and through the nail plate. Although 100% poration allowed for the greatest amount of drug delivered to the nail plate, the nails that were 40% to 70% porated reached a steady-state drug delivery rate and may be a more ideal option for rapid, deep penetration of various drug therapies to the nail bed. Of note, 100% poration through the nail may compromise the barrier function, whereas 40% to 70% poration allows better penetration of a model compound through the nail plate, without compromising much nail barrier function. In another study by Tsai and colleagues,[23] it was shown that fractional CO_2 laser can also be used to successfully porate the nail plate, resulting in enhanced drug delivery.

Chemical

Chemical enhancements include the use of thiols, sulfites, hydrogen peroxide, urea, water, keratinolytic enzyme, and keratolytic enhancers. In a study by Joshi and colleagues,[24] it was found that thioglycolic acid enhanced the permeation of a compounded drug through the nail plate. This was achieved through the sulfhydryl group in the thioglycolic acid, which can cleave the numerous disulfide bonds in keratin of the nail plate. Comparatively, a lacquer formulation without the thioglycolic acid was not able to penetrate as deep as the formulation with the thioglycolic acid, nor could it diffusely spread throughout the nail plate. Therefore, it can be postulated that formulas with thiols will have better penetration through the nail plate, and thus, a better therapeutic outcome. Further studies on other chemical enhancements are necessary to evaluate their efficacy in enhancing topical penetration.

ANTIFUNGAL MEDICATIONS SPECIFICALLY FORMULATED TO PENETRATE THE NAIL

There are specific drugs that have been developed that show adequate nail penetration. Tavaborole topical solution 5% exhibits both chemical and physical properties that make it useable as a topical treatment for onychomycosis, including a low-molecular-weight and boron chemistry. A study by Coronado and colleagues[25] was done in ex vivo human fingernails to determine whether there is a difference in tavaborole's activity in the presence of keratin. Tavaborole was fungicidal against T rubrum and T mentagrophytes. The penetration of 5% tavaborole topical treatment through human fingernails was about 40 times greater than 8% ciclopirox nail lacquer treatment after 14 days.

Efinaconazole topical solution 10% also exhibits a smaller molecular weight that allows penetration through the nail plate compared with other topical medications and is hydrophilic. Efinaconazole has also been found to penetrate the nail better than ciclopirox and amorolfine because of its lower affinity for keratin. Lower keratin-binding affinity allows it to penetrate the nail plate and approach the nail bed where the dermatophyte infection began. The risk in recurrence of disease is lowered by maintaining levels of drugs on the nails. Further research needs to be done to investigate if it is possible to maintain efinaconazole levels for an extended course to attain the decrease in risk.[16]

SUMMARY

Topical treatments for nail diseases must be specially formulated because of the thick nail plate barrier and the possible drug-binding affinity for keratin. Antifungal medications like efinaconazole and tavaborole have shown favorable use because of their low molecular weight and hydrophilicity, which leads to better transit across the nail plate. Recent research has focused on mechanical debridement to thin the nail plate directly and physical enhancements to increase polarity for penetration into the nail bed. Chemical keratolytics have been shown to increase drug penetration through the nail plate by cleaving the disulfide bonds of keratin, but further investigation is required to determine the efficacy of keratolytics drugs in combination with current antifungal medications.

CLINICS CARE POINTS

- It is beneficial to treat any nail condition early in the disease process with topical drugs that do not bind keratin or do not have a high affinity to keratin.

- Tavaborole topical solution 5% exhibits both chemical and physical properties that make it useable as a topical treatment for onychomycosis, including a low-molecular-weight and boron chemistry.

- Efinaconazole's lower keratin-binding affinity allows it to penetrate the nail plate and approach the nail bed where the dermatophyte infection began.

REFERENCES

1. Barron JN. The structure and function of the skin of the hand. Hand 1970; 2(2):93–6.
2. Murdan S. Drug delivery to the nail following topical application. Int J Pharm 2002;236(1–2):1–26.
3. Elewski BE. Onychomycosis: treatment, quality of life, and economic issues. Am J Clin Dermatol 2000;1(1):415–29.
4. Foster KW, Ghannoum MA, Elewski BE. Epidemiologic surveillance of cutaneous fungal infection in the United States from 1999 to 2002. J Am Acad Dermatol 2004;50(5):748–52.
5. Elewski BE. Onychomycosis: pathogenesis, diagnosis, and management. Clin Microbiol Rev 1998;11(3):415–29.
6. Scher RK. Onychomycosis: a significant medical disorder. J Am Acad Dermatol 1996;35(3):S2–5.
7. Henseler T, Christophers E. Psoriasis of early and late onset: characterization of two types of psoriasis vulgaris. J Am Acad Dermatol 1985;13(3):450–6.
8. De Berker D. Diagnosis and management of nail psoriasis. Dermatol Ther 2002; 15(2):165–72.
9. Saner MV, Kulkarni AD, Pardeshi CV. Insights into drug delivery across the nail plate barrier. J Drug Target 2014;22(9):769–89.
10. Zaias N. Psoriasis of the nail: a clinical-pathologic study. Arch Dermatol 1969; 99(5):567–79.
11. Hui X, Baker SJ, Wester RC, et al. In vitro penetration of a novel oxaborole antifungal (AN2690) into the human nail plate. J Pharm Sci 2007;96(10):2622–31.
12. McAuley WJ, Jones SA, Traynor MJ, et al. An investigation of how fungal infection influences drug penetration through onychomycosis patient's nail plates. Eur J Pharm Biopharm 2016;102:178–84.
13. Krönauer C, Gfesser M, Ring J, et al. Transonychial water loss in healthy and diseased nails. Acta Derm Venereol 2001;81(3):175–7.
14. Walters KA, Flynn GL, Marvel JR. Physicochemical characterization of the human nail: solvent effects on the permeation of homologous alcohols. J Pharm Pharmacol 1985;37(11):771–5.
15. Palmeri A, Pichini S, Pacifici R, et al. Drugs in nails. Clin Pharmacokinet 2000; 38(2):95–110.
16. Sakamoto M, Sugimoto N, Kawabata H, et al. Transungual delivery of efinaconazole: its deposition in the nail of onychomycosis patients and in vitro fungicidal activity in human nails. J Drugs Dermatol 2014;13(11):1388–92.

17. Hao J, Li SK. Transungual iontophoretic transport of polar neutral and positively charged model permeants: effects of electrophoresis and electroosmosis. J Pharm Sci 2008;97(2):893–905.

18. Kobayashi Y, Miyamoto M, Sugibayashi K, et al. Drug permeation through the three layers of the human nail plate. J Pharm Pharmacol 1999;51:271–8.

19. Baran R, Hay RJ, Garduno JI. Review of antifungal therapy and the severity index for assessing onychomycosis: part I. J Dermatolog Treat 2008;19(2):72–81.

20. Dutet J, Delgado-Charro MB. In vivo transungual iontophoresis: effect of DC current application on ionic transport and on transonychial water loss. J Control Release 2009;140(2):117–25.

21. Dutet J, Delgado-Charro MB. Transungual iontophoresis of lithium and sodium: effect of pH and co-ion competition on cationic transport numbers. J Control Release 2010;144(2):168–74.

22. Vanstone S, Cordery SF, Stone JM, et al. Precise laser poration to control drug delivery into and through human nail. J Control Release 2017;268:72–7.

23. Tsai MT, Tsai TY, Shen SC, et al. Evaluation of laser-assisted trans-nail drug delivery with optical coherence tomography. Sensors (Switzerland) 2016;16(12):2111.

24. Joshi M, Sharma V, Pathak K. Matrix based system of isotretinoin as nail lacquer to enhance transungal delivery across human nail plate. Int J Pharm 2015;478(1): 268–77.

25. Coronado DB, Merchant MPharm T, Chanda S, et al. In vitro nail penetration and antifungal activity of tavaborole, a boron-based pharmaceutical. J Drugs Dermatol 2015;14(6):609–14.

Plantar Psoriasis
A Review of the Literature

Michael Romani, DPM, Garrett Biela, DPM, Kalen Farr, DPM,
Ryan Lazar, DPM, Marcus Duval, DPM, Victoria Trovillion, DPM,
Tracey C. Vlahovic, DPM*

KEYWORDS

- Palmoplantar psoriasis • Plantar psoriasis • Palmoplantar pustulosis • Phototherapy
- Apremilast • Biologic therapy • Combination therapy

KEY POINTS

- Topical treatment options are considered first line therapy for plantar psoriasis and consist of topical corticosteroids and topical non-corticosteroids.
- Phototherapy, systemic agents, and biologic agents may be used once topical therapy has been used and/or failed.
- There is no consensus on treatment for plantar psoriasis, so the practitioner must consider risk vs benefit and the quality of life that is impacted when choosing therapy regimens.

INTRODUCTION

Psoriasis is an inflammatory disorder of the skin, varying in distribution and severity, but chronic in nature. Plaques are observed on an erythematous, scaly base in generalized psoriasis, whereas the less common palmoplantar psoriasis (PP) variant may present with plaques, pustules, or a combination of both occurring on the palms of the hands and soles of the feet. The localized distribution of pustules on the palmar and plantar surface can distinguish PP from generalized psoriasis.[1,2] Psoriasis is a clinical diagnosis, and for PP, the palmar surface of the hands should always be checked when the plantar surface is involved to refine the diagnosis. Psoriatic episodes can be triggered by a multitude of events, ranging from infection and trauma to smoking and stress[2] (**Fig. 1**).

Because of weight bearing on the plantar surface of the foot, PP can be exceptionally debilitating and excruciating. Although the body surface area involved is relatively small compared with generalized plaque psoriasis, the plantar surface distributes the entirety of the body weight with each step, causing greater irritation and worsening of

Conflict of Interest: none of the authors have any financial interests to disclose for this article.
Temple University School of Podiatric Medicine, 148 North 8th Street, Philadelphia, PA 19107, USA
* Corresponding author.
E-mail address: traceyv@temple.edu

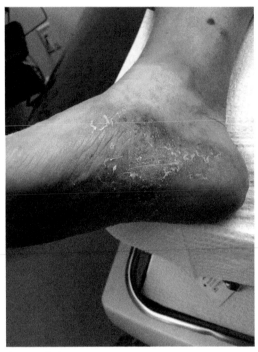

Fig. 1. Plantar pustular psoriasis.

the condition, known as the Koebner phenomenon.[3] PP can have a negative impact both on quality of life and overall psychological well-being (**Fig. 2**).

Palmoplantar pustulosis (PPP) is believed to be a genetic variant of psoriasis. Some argue that there are histopathological similarities between PP and PPP. However, other literature suggests the 2 are entirely different, although the distinction is still not well understood.[4]

There are several treatments options for PP. The general first-line therapy is an integrated use of topical corticosteroids, retinoids, vitamin D analogues, and/or keratolytics. Phototherapy is also a treatment option, with outcomes demonstrating an extended remission period compared with other treatments. In cases of severe PP, systemic or biological therapy are typically considered as primary therapy.[5] Although there are several treatment options for PP, there currently is no consensus on a specific therapy regimen. Finding a therapy that effectively clears the lesions with minimal adverse effects or contraindications proves to be a challenge, as even a highly potent therapy regimen has variable results between individual patients. This article reviews the literature to determine if a potential standard of care for PP exists (**Fig. 3**).

TOPICAL TREATMENT OPTIONS

Topical treatments such as corticosteroids, retinoids, vitamin D analogues, salicylic acid, and emollients are considered first-line therapy to manage PP. In 80% of patients diagnosed with PP, topical steroids are the primary treatment option because of the potent antiinflammatory, immunosuppressive, and antiproliferative properties.[3,6] Topical steroids are the preferred initial treatment compared with systemic steroids due to the lessened adverse effects with local application and the possibility of systemic steroids precipitating a worsened presentation.[7] However, prolonged exposure

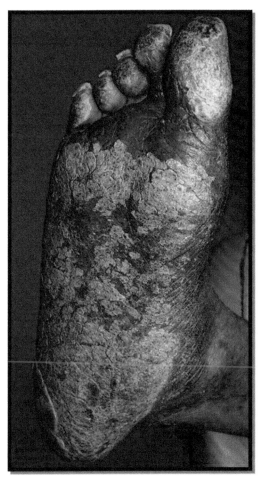

Fig. 2. Plantar plaque psoriasis.

of steroids over a large surface area can cause skin atrophy and possible systemic absorption, among other characteristic side effects. To minimize potential adverse effects and increase efficacy, treatment should incorporate combination therapy and cycling of topical steroids in order to have a steroid sparing effect.[8]

Tazarotene, a topical retinoid, is a valuable adjunct to treating PP by decreasing the rate of differentiation and production of keratinocytes. Tazarotene can also be used as an alternative to steroids if the side effects of the steroids are too severe.[3] However, evidence indicates dual use of topical tazarotene, and a topical steroid can decrease the skin atrophy caused by the steroid, as well as produce a synergistic effect, allowing the use of a lowered dose that is equally effective.[9] For PP, the combination of a topical retinoid and a topical steroid could assist in lessening the thickened plaques often seen. The drawback of topical retinoid use is the high occurrence of irritation; therefore, it should be applied sparingly, especially around lesions.[10] The adverse effects of topical steroids and retinoids can potentially be avoided with emollients. Emollients create a protective layer over the epidermis, increasing hydration and subsequently lowering the possibility of erythema and scaling.[11] Studies demonstrate that mixing emollients with betamethasone, a class 1 corticosteroid, can increase the

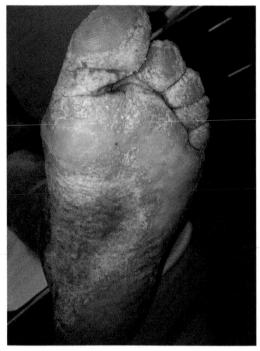

Fig. 3. Patient before phototherapy.

efficacy of the steroid as well as reduce the number of applications to achieve desired effects.[12]

Keratolytics, such as salicylic acid, in low concentrations are useful in lessening hyperkeratotic scales involved in PP.[13] Utilization of keratolytics is particularly advantageous as combination therapy with a steroid or retinoid to improve absorption for maximal effectiveness. However, keratolytics should not be used with vitamin D analogues or ultraviolet (UV) ray therapy.[3]

Vitamin D analogues, known as calcipotriene and calcitriol, inhibit keratinocyte production and are therefore another acceptable adjunct treatment of PP with topical steroids.[8] Previous studies found that vitamin D analogues and steroids used simultaneously have improved effects in comparison to monotherapy, as well as decreased side effects due to the reduced dose of the steroid.[6]

Although topical treatments are a suitable first-line therapy for PP, the length of application and adherence to application can be discouraging to patients, especially with incomplete clearance of the lesions. Also, the thickened stratum corneum of the plantar skin may limit absorption; therefore, choosing the correct vehicle for application is imperative. The most successful therapy is an individualized combination of topicals for each patient to limit adverse effects and increase effectiveness. In addition, clearly written and verbal instructions for the patient should be provided because the regimen requires compliance over an extended period of time.[8]

PHOTOTHERAPY/PHOTOCHEMOTHERAPY

Phototherapy is a frequently used therapy for psoriasis; however, there is currently no defined regimen of treatment strength or duration for PP. There are various ways to deliver radiation therapy to the skin, but the most common are using narrowband UVB[14] or a combination of UVA with a photosensitizer agent such as psoralen.[8,15,16] One aspect all phototherapy studies demonstrate is the longer periods of remission compared with the traditional topical medication treatments for PP. Thus, phototherapy is often used after failed treatments of topical medications.

A study by Gianfaldoni and colleagues evaluated PPP treatment with narrowband UVB therapy at 308 nm, to reduce collateral damage on nonaffected skin. This treatment was performed twice a week for the 4 weeks and subsequently once a week for the next 4 weeks. Duration of treatment started at 15 seconds for the first session and increased 5 seconds thereafter. After 16 sessions, the patient achieved complete remission in the affected areas and remained clear through 12 weeks of evaluation with no treatment. A major advantage to UVB therapy, as opposed to UVA, is decreased skin penetrance, resulting in little to no risk of future skin cancer development, and no chemical adjuvants are required.

In contrast, a study by Fritsch and colleagues (1978) tested the effects of PUVA therapy (UVA radiation with Psoralen) augmented with another photosensitizer methoxsalen and compared it with administration of standard PUVA therapy, as well as administration of an oral retinoic acid derivative only. The study discovered that the addition of methoxsalen resulted in a 30% to 50% decrease in the total duration and number of treatments (mean of 10 irradiation in 17 days), as well as a 75% decrease in the total cumulative UVA energy applied to the patient compared with traditional PUVA therapy. This significant reduction in exposure and treatment time is considerably more beneficial and safer to the patient. Although PUVA therapy with methoxsalen has been proved a very effective method, the authors acknowledge that there is still the long-term risk of developing skin cancers.

Overall, evidence suggests the use of phototherapy/photochemotherapy is an effective method of treating PP as a first-line treatment or after the failure of topical treatments (**Fig. 4**).

SYSTEMIC TREATMENT

Systemic treatments for psoriasis are often used once a patient fails multiple treatment options such as first-line topical or phototherapy. PP and PPP are very difficult to treat in general and often cause functional disability due to lesion location.

Multiple case studies illustrate an effective systemic treatment of PP and PPP, but they often lack a large sample size. In a retrospective study, 45 of 62 patients with PP and 34 of 52 patients with PPP required systemic treatment after failed improvement with topical agents. Many of these patients also required multiple systemic treatments. Marked improvement (>75% area cleared) occurred in 52.9% of the patients with PP treated with systemic retinoids, PUVA, methotrexate, cyclosporine, or a combination of these drugs. Marked improvement occurred in 56.6% of the patients with PPP treated with systemic retinoids, colchicine, PUVA, methotrexate, cyclosporine, or some combination of these drugs.[17] This retrospective study helps illustrate the difficulty in treating PP/PPP, while noting the importance of combination therapy to see significant improvement in the patient's condition.

One of the most used systemic drugs for PP, outside of women of child-bearing age is the oral retinoid, acitretin.[18] Acitretin combined with PUVA is often the retinoid of choice in patients with PP/PPP.[3] However, acitretin has known teratogenic effects and systemic abnormalities associated with its use. A double-blind, randomized, placebo-controlled study was performed using liarozole, a retinoic acid metabolism-blocking drug and aromatase inhibitor, to search for a safer alternative. This study

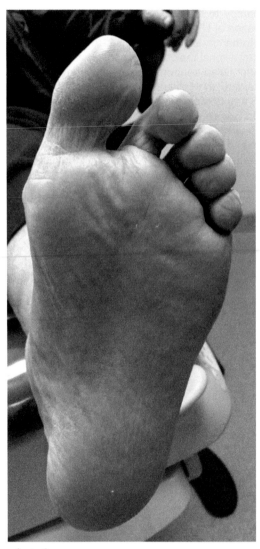

Fig. 4. Patient after phototherapy.

prescribed 75 mg, 2 times per day for 12 weeks in 15 actively smoking patients of both sexes, aged 18 to 70 years. Data were recorded at weeks 0, 2, 4, 8, and 12 using multiple scores based on erythema, pustules, desquamation, and percent area of palms/soles affected. Side effects and regimen compliance were also monitored. There were significantly lower scores in the liarozole patients when compared with the placebo. Four of the seven liarozole patients saw greater than 70% improvement after 12 weeks, whereas only one of the placebo patients saw such improvement. No patients withdrew from side effects related to retinoic acid levels, and only 2 of 7 liarozole patients experienced self-limiting severe cheilitis, with no abnormalities in hematology or biochemistry found.[19] The results of this study confirm the efficacy of systemic treatment in severe PP, while providing promising results for larger scale studies looking into safer alternative treatment options.

Finally, a more recent study was done on the efficacy and safety of apremilast (Ote-zla), a phosphodiesterase-4 inhibitor. In the double-blind, randomized, placebo trial, patients were prescribed 30 mg, twice per day for 16 weeks. Data were recorded using the PPPGA scale based on severity from 0 (clear) to 4 (severe, dark red). Of the 1431 total patients pooled, 427 members had PP, with 144 of the cases being moderate or severe (3–4 PPPGA). After 16 weeks, 48% of the apremilast group and 27% of the placebo group improved from a 3 to 4 PPPGA to a 0 to 1 PPGA. In the mild (PPPGA 1–2) pool, 46% of apremilast and 25% of placebo patients improved to a completely clear, or 0, PPPGA. No serious systemic side effects such as cellulitis occurred; however, greater than 5% of the apremilast patients experienced diarrhea, nausea/vomiting, headaches, upper respiratory infections, or nasopharyngitis.[20] Bissonnette and colleagues' data suggest that apremilast can be effective in patients with both mild and severe PP. Previous studies illustrated the importance of combination therapy in PP/PPP,[17] and data from this study may be useful in incorporating apremilast into future regimens (**Figs. 5** and **6**).

Although there is no definitive choice for a single systemic agent in the treatment of PP, there is promising data on their importance in more severe cases. In these cases,

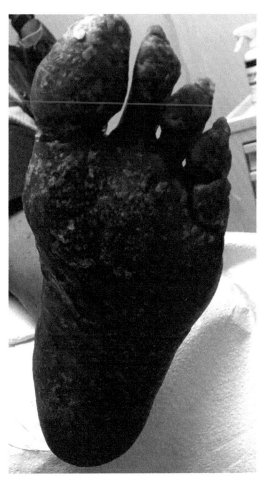

Fig. 5. Baseline before apremilast therapy.

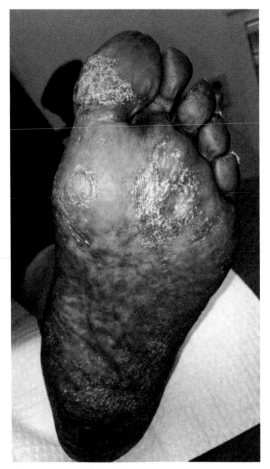

Fig. 6. Patient after 30 days of apremilast therapy.

systemic agents, such as an oral retinoid or PDIE-4 inhibitor, have been shown to be both effective and safe. Future studies may be able to help expand on the Adışen and colleagues study and determine a definitive combination of these agents.

BIOLOGICS

The use of biologics for the treatment of psoriasis is relatively new in comparison to its other indications such as for rheumatoid arthritis.[21] Currently, the American Academy of Dermatology recommends biologics as third- or fourth-line therapies, to be used in conjunction with other medications.[22,23] The recommendation to reserve biological therapy is due to the potential for inducing pustular flares and the high financial burden.[24,25] Studies show the risk of flares is reduced using continuous dosing versus intermittent treatment with the medication.[26]

Apart from the reported flares, biologics are well tolerated and "pose little risk of end organ damage" when compared with other systemic agents such as cyclosporine and methotrexate.[22,27] Despite this low risk, it is important to consider the patient's comorbidities and severity of psoriasis before starting a biologic.[22] Clinical practice guidelines recommend looking for human immunodeficiency virus, hepatitis B, hepatitis

C, tuberculosis, or any other granulomatous infection and malignancy.[5,28] These comorbidities can be reactivated following therapy with biologics.[29]

PP is particularly difficult to treat, and patients suffer a disproportionate amount of pain due to the lesions impairing walking and manual dexterity.[30,31] Some biologics have had better results in PP than other treatment options.[30] Ustekinumab (Stelara) is a recently approved biologic used to treat plaque psoriasis by inhibiting both interleukin-12 (IL-12) and IL-23, which stops the inflammatory cascade.[32,33] Ustekinumab has also shown to be just as effective for PP after other conservative treatments failed.[34] Similarly, secukinumab is an antiinterleukin 17A antibody that also is particularly effective in patients with PP.[31]

Few comparisons have been made between biologics and other treatment options.[21] There is, however, some insight into the cost efficiency of biologics, as treatment can be expensive. The high cost has prompted insurance companies to enact rigid eligibility criteria that patients need to meet, such as previously failing improvement with topical or phototherapies.[25,35] A study by Chi and colleagues (2014) compared the commonly used biologics for psoriasis and determined that adalimumab, a tumor necrosis factor alpha inhibitor, was the most cost-efficient. Cost efficiency is particularly important in psoriasis, as it is a condition that cannot be cured and requires long-term treatment.[35,36] Despite the cost, treatment with biologics remain an effective second-tier agent for the treatment of PP.[5,37]

SUMMARY

Currently, there is no consensus on a standard of care for PP due to the challenge of achieving remission in a safe, effective manner. Evidence shows combination therapy is always more effective than monotherapy in both clearance of the lesions and improvement in quality of life.

Topicals are generally safer and more cost-efficient for long-term use, making it an excellent first-line treatment option. Patients should begin with a combination of a topical steroid, vitamin D analogue, and emollient. Long-term use of this topical therapy may require cycling of the steroid to avoid adverse effects. If the patient suffers from the plaque form of PP, salicylic acid can be considered in place of the vitamin D analogue to assist the steroids in penetrating excess scale.

Phototherapy, particularly using narrowband UVB, is also a safe treatment option that should be used in addition to topical therapy, especially for moderate-to-severe cases. Evidence shows PUVA + methoxsalen improves remission duration. However, due to the uncertain long-term risk of skin cancer, consideration should be taken to limiting phototherapy to initial treatment and intermittent flares. PP is particularly difficult to treat, and because of the significant impact on quality of life, therapy often resorts to systemic treatment in addition to topical/phototherapy. Apremilast is a successful adjunct to therapy with mild adverse effects.

Biologics such as adalimumab are effective; however, because of the expense of the drug for long-term use, it is often not a primary treatment option. Special attention should be taken if the patient has a severe chronic infection or malignancy, as biologics are contraindicated. An ideal candidate for biologics is someone who has moderate-to-severe PP, no chronic infection, and no history of malignancy.

Therapy for PP should be approached as a stepwise gradient beginning with topicals and progressing to systemics. Each progression in therapy should build on the previous because combination therapy has consistently proved to be more effective. As always, review of the patient's severity of condition, health status, and lifestyle is needed to individualize therapy for the best patient care.

CLINICS CARE POINTS

- Combination therapy with topical medications or topical plus phototherapy or systemic medications seem to have better efficacy than monotherapy.
- Step-wise therapy is recommended when building a treatment protocol, with each new therapy building on what has been given previously.
- Plantar psoriasis is most commonly a clinical diagnosis; so it is important to check the palmar hands for skin lesions and ask the patient if there is a history of psoriasis or any other skin rashes on the body.

REFERENCES

1. Meier M, Sheth PB. Clinical spectrum and severity of psoriasis. Curr Probl Dermatol 2009;38:1–20.
2. Farley E, Masrour S, McKey J, et al. Palmoplantar psoriasis: a phenotypical and clinical review with introduction of a new quality-of-life assessment tool. J Am Acad Dermatol 2009;60:1024–31.
3. Engin B, Aşkın Ö, Tüzün Y. Palmoplantar psoriasis. Clin Dermatol 2017;35 1: 19–27.
4. Naik HB, Cowen EW. Autoinflammatory pustular neutrophilic diseases. Dermatol Clin 2013;31:405–25.
5. Menter A, Gottlieb A, Feldman SR, et al. Guidelines of care for the management of psoriasis and psoriatic arthritis: section 1. Overview of psoriasis and guidelines of care for the treatment of psoriasis with biologics. J Am Acad Dermatol 2008;58: 826–50.
6. Menter A, Korman NJ, Elmets CA, et al. Guidelines of care for the management of psoriasis and psoriatic arthritis: section 3. Guidelines of care for the management and treatment of psoriasis with topical therapies. J AM Acad Dermatol 2009;61: 451–85.
7. Menter A, Korman NJ, Elmets CA, et al. Guidelines of care for the management of psoriasis and psoriatic arthritis Section 6. Guidelines of care for the treatment of psoriasis and psoriatic arthritis: case-based presentations and evidence-based conclusions. Am Acad Dermatol 2011;65:137–74.
8. Menter A, Korman NJ, Elmets CA, et al. Guidelines of care for the management of psoriasis and psoriatic arthritis: section 6. Guidelines of care for the treatment of psoriasis and psoriatic arthritis: case-based presentation and evidence based conclusions. J Am Acad Dermatol 2011;65:137–74.
9. Handa S. Newer trends in the management of psoriasis at difficult to treat locations: scalp, palmoplantar disease and nails. Indian J Dermatol Venereol Leprol 2010;76:634–44.
10. Umezawa Y, Nakagawa H, Tamaki K. Phase III clinical study of maxacal- citol ointment in patients with palmoplantar pustulosis: a randomized, double-blind, placebo-controlled trial. J Dermatol 2016;43:288–93.
11. Mehta BH, Amladi ST. Evaluation of topical 0.1% tazarotene cream in the treatment of palmoplantar psoriasis: an observer-blinded randomized controlled study. Indian J Dermatol 2011;56:40–3.
12. Watsky KL, Freije L, Leneveu MC, et al. Water-in-oil emollients as steroid-sparing adjunctive therapy in the treatment of psoriasis. Cutis 1992;50:383–6.

13. Rim JH, Jo SJ, Park JY, et al. Electrical measure- ment of moisturizing effect on skin hydration and barrier function in psoriasis patients. Clin Exp Dermatol 2005;30:409–13.
14. Duman D. Topical treatments of psoriasis. Turkiye Klinikleri J Dermatol Spec Top 2008;1:55–62.
15. Sumila M, Notter M, Itin P, et al. Long-term results of radiotherapy in patients with chronic palmo-plantar eczema or psoriasis. Strahlenther Onkol 2008;184:218–23.
16. Fritsch PO, Honigsmann H, Jaschke E, et al. Augmentation of oral methoxsalen photochemotherapy with an oral retinoic acid derivative. J Investig Dermatol 1978;70(4):178–82.
17. Gianfaldoni S, Tchernev G, Wollina U, et al. Pustular palmoplantar psoriasis suc- cessfully treated with Nb-UVB monochromatic excimer light: a case-report. Open Access Maced J Med Sci 2017;5(4):462–6.
18. Adışen E, Tekin O, Gülekon A, et al. A retrospective analysis of treatment re- sponses of palmoplantar psoriasis in 114 patients. J Eur Acad Dermatol Venereol 2009;23:814–9.
19. Chalmers R, Hollis S, Leonardi-Bee J, et al. Interventions for chronic palmoplantar pustulosis. Cochrane Database Syst Rev 2006;(1):CD001433.
20. Bhushan M, Burden A, MCelhone K, et al. Oral liarozole in the treatment of palmo- plantar pustular psoriasis: a randomized, double-blind, placebo-controlled study. Br J Dermatol 2001;145:546–53.
21. Bissonnette R, Pariser DM, Wasel NR, et al. Apremilast, an oral phosphodiesterase-4 inhibitor, in the treatment of palmoplantar psoriasis: results of a pooled analysis from phase II PSOR-005 and phase III Efficacy and Safety Trial Evaluating the Effects of Apremilast in Psoriasis (ESTEEM) clinical trials in patients with moderate to severe psoriasis. J Am Acad Dermatol 2016;75(1): 99–105.
22. Hsu S, Papp K, Lebwohl MG, et al. Consensus guidelines for the management of plaque psoriasis. Arch Dermatol 2012;148:95–102.
23. Weisman S, Pollack CR, Gottschalk RW. Psoriasis disease severity measures: comparing efficacy of treatments for severe psoriasis. J Dermatolog Treat 2003;14:158–65.
24. Michaelsson G, Kajermo U, Michaelsson A, et al. Infliximab can precipitate as well as worsen palmoplantar pustulosis: possible linkage to the expression of tumour necrosis factor- alpha in the normal palmar eccrine sweat duct? Br J Der- matol 2005;153:1243–4.
25. Anis AH, Bansback N, Sizto S, et al. Economic evaluation of biologic therapies for the treatment of moderate to severe psoriasis in the United States. J Dermatol Treat 2011;22(2):65–74.
26. Reich K, Wozel G, Zheng H, et al. Efficacy and safety of inflix- imab as continuous or intermittent therapy in patients with moderate-to-severe plaque psoriasis: re- sults of a random- ized, long-term extension trial (RESTORE2). Br J Dermatol 2013;168:1325–34.
27. Tyring S, Gordon KB, Poulin Y, et al. Long-term safety and efficacy of 50mg of eta- nercept twice weekly in patients with psoriasis. Arch Dermatol 2007;143:719–26.
28. Smith CH, Anstey AV, Barker JN, et al. British Association of Dermatologists' guidelines for biologic interventions for psoriasis 2009. Br J Dermatol 2009; 161:987–1019.
29. Pathirana D, Ormerod AD, Saiag P, et al. European S3-guide- lines on the sys- temic treatment of psoriasis vulgaris. J Eur Acad Dermatol Venereol 2009; 23(Suppl 2):1–70.

30. Au SC, Madani A, Alhaddad M, et al. Comparison of the efficacy of biologics versus conventional systemic therapies in the treatment of psoriasis at a comprehensive psoriasis care center. J Drugs Dermatol 2013;12:861–6.
31. Gottlieb A, Sullivan J, van Doorn M, et al. Secukinumab shows significant efficacy in palmoplantar psoriasis: results from GESTURE, a randomized controlled trial. J Am Acad Dermatol 2016;76(1):70–80. Available at: www.sciencedirect.com/science/article/pii/S0190962216306120.
32. Tang C, Chen S, Qlan H, et al. Interleukin-23: as a drug target for autoimmune inflammatory disease. Immunology 2012;135:112–24.
33. Leonardi CL, Kimball AB, Papp KA, et al. Efficacy and safety of ustekinumab, a human interleukin- 12/23 monoclonal antibody, in patients with psoriasis: 76-week results from a randomized, double-blind, placebo-controlled trial (PHOENIX 1). Lancet 2008;371:1665–74.
34. Vlahovic TC, James MM. Ustekinumab in the treatment of moderate to severe lower extremity psoriasis: a case series. The Foot and Ankle Online Journal 2012;5(11):1. Available at: faoj.org/2012/11/01/ustekinumab-in-the-treatment-of-moderate-to-severe-lower-extremity-psoriasis-a-case-series/.
35. Chi CC, Wang SH. Efficacy and cost-efficacy of biologic therapies for moderate to severe psoriasis: a meta-analysis and cost-efficacy analysis using the Intention-to-treat principle. Biomed Res Int 2014;2014:862851. Available at: www.hindawi.com/journals/bmri/2014/862851/.
36. Colombo GL, Di Matteo S, Peris K, et al. A cost-utility analysis of etanercept for the treatment of moderate-to-severe psoriasis in Italy. Clinicoeco Outcomes Res 2009;1(1):53–9.
37. Shah VV, Lee EB, Reddy S, et al. Comparison of guidelines for the Use of TNF inhibitors for psoriasis in the United States, Canada, europe and the United Kingdom: a critical appraisal and comprehensive review. J Dermatol Treat 2018;29(6):586–92.

Use of Biologics in the Treatment of Moderate-to-Severe Plantar Psoriasis

Josh Ekladios, DPM, Jason Jolliffe, DPM, Shalin Panchigar, DPM,
Rafay Qureshi, DPM, Ankita Shete, DPM, Jason Wellner, DPM,
Tracey C. Vlahovic, DPM*

KEYWORDS

- Psoriasis • Interleukin • Biologics • Inflammatory • Monoclonal antibodies
- Cytokine

KEY POINTS

- Lower extremity psoriasis can manifest as skin lesions, nail dystrophy, and/or arthritis. Biologic therapy is useful in treating these manifestations.
- The usefulness of biologics lies in their targeted binding and inhibition of inflammatory mediators, such as interferon gamma (IFNg), interleukins (IL), and tumor necrosis factor alpha (TNFa), all of which have been linked to psoriatic flares.
- Psoriasis is a chronic autoimmune disease that causes systemic inflammation. Besides physical pain and disability, patients suffer emotional stress from its effect on their visual appearance.

INTRODUCTION

Psoriasis is a chronic inflammatory skin condition that affects nearly 7.5 million Americans.[1] Symptoms range from dermatologic issues such as dry, cracked skin that may itch or burn to thick, pitted nails. Symptoms can also present systemically in the form of fever, chills, muscle weakness, and associated arthritis.[2] Physical examination findings, particularly the location of lesions, vary from patient to patient and subtype to subtype. Plaque psoriasis, which comprises nearly 80% of cases, presents classically as red plaques covered with silvery scales and can occur on any surface of the body.[3] Psoriasis is not an infectious disease; rather, it is an autoimmune disorder that leads to uncontrolled cutaneous, bowel, or synovial inflammation.[4]

Palmoplantar pustulosis (PPP) refers to a subtype of pustular psoriasis that appears on the palms of the hands and soles of the feet, predominantly in female patients aged between 20 and 60 years . PPP is readily identified by its hallmark feature, pus-filled

Conflict of Interest: none of the authors have any financial interests to disclose for this article.
Temple University School of Podiatric Medicine, 148 N 8th Street, Philadelphia, PA 19107, USA
* Corresponding author.
E-mail address: traceyv@temple.edu

formations atop erythematous skin lesions, which people wrongly assume are contagious. When PPP or plaque psoriasis is present on the plantar feet, it is considered a moderate presentation even though the surface area is not as large as the rest of the body. Constant irritation of these pustules or plaques when walking or standing can be debilitating if it significantly interferes with a patient's activities of daily living. Toenails and the small joints of the foot can also be affected by psoriasis. Biological therapy is a promising treatment to assist the lower extremity psoriasis patient from these manifestations.

Considering the tremendous variation in demographics, clinical presentations, and treatment response of patients with psoriasis, a high number of pharmacotherapeutic agents have been developed in an attempt to alleviate symptoms.[1] Treatment proves difficult because the course of the disease depends on both environmental and genetic factors, as well as most cases being recalcitrant to single-agent therapy.[5] Among the treatment options available to physicians are topical corticosteroids, ultraviolet light phototherapy, vitamin D analogues, nonaromatic moisturizers, oral phosphodiesterase-4 inhibitors, and injectable or intravenous biological drugs. The usefulness of biologics lies in their targeted binding and inhibition of inflammatory mediators, such as interferon gamma (IFNγ), interleukins (IL), and tumor necrosis factor alpha (TNFα), all of which have been linked to psoriatic flares.[6] The main limitation in research of biologics is the complicated interplay between these various mediators. However, clinicians continue to use these therapies due to their promising effects in controlling and treating moderate-to-severe psoriatic symptoms.

CLASSES OF BIOLOGICAL AGENTS
Interleukin-23 Inhibitors

It is well known that IL-12 and IL-23 are effective target sites for treating inflammatory skin disorders. However, new studies suggest that IL-23 plays a bigger role in cytokine generation and autoimmunity in psoriasis through its regulation of Th17 effector cells.[7,8] Th17 cells secrete IL-17 that has been shown to activate memory T cells and recruit macrophages to sites of infection. Monoclonal antibodies that target the p40 subunit found in both IL-12 and IL-23 actually show a higher selectivity for IL-23 than IL-12.[8] This increased selectivity could be a promising lead in the development of new biologics for psoriasis that specifically target the IL-23-Th17 axis.

Relatively new to the market, guselkumab is an IL-23 inhibitor that shows great promise in treating psoriasis and psoriatic arthritis. In a phase III trial, guselkumab was tested to see if IL-23 inhibitors alone are effective in treating psoriasis. A single dose of 10, 100, or 300 mg were given to patients.[9] After 24 weeks, patients showed signs of 50%, 60%, and 100% improvement, respectively, but a larger trial needs to be done to confirm efficacy and safety. Another phase III trial was conducted comparing guselkumab with adalimumab in patients with moderate-to-severe psoriasis. Although both biologics had increased incidence of upper respiratory infection, headache, and nasopharyngitis, adalimumab caused more frequent injection site reaction and led to one cardiovascular event.[10] Guselkumab showed greater efficacy in treatment of psoriasis as well as less safety concerns as compared with adalimumab. Therefore, IL-23 inhibitors such as guselkumab may be a long-term and well-tolerated treatment option for patients with moderate-to-severe psoriasis.

Interleukin-12/23 Inhibitors

Ustekinumab is a human immunoglobulin G (IgG) 1 kappa monoclonal antibody that binds the p40 subunit found in IL-12 and IL-23.[11] Because these cytokines play a central role in the recruitment of various immune cells, inhibiting them from activating receptor complexes prevents a myriad of downstream effects.[12] IL-12 is produced by dendritic cells, macrophages, and neutrophils in response to antigens and drives the differentiation of Th1 cells. In addition to producing inflammatory mediators such as IFNγ and TNFα, Th1 cells shepherd T cells to the skin surface via cutaneous lymphocyte antigen, a proposed mechanism for skin lesion development in autoimmune diseases such as psoriasis.[13] Together, IL-12 and IL-23 work synergistically to produce additional immune responses via natural killer cells and specific T-cell subsets.[14]

Ustekinumab is a successful treatment of many autoimmune diseases. Because biopsies of psoriatic skin lesions show increased levels of IL-12, IL-23, and their downstream products, it can be used in plaque psoriasis and psoriatic arthritis.[15] It is administered by subcutaneous injection in doses of 45 or 90 mg and has a half-life of 15 to 32 days. After initial dosing, patients receive a second injection at 4 weeks and then every 12 weeks thereafter.[12,14] Clinical efficacy of ustekinumab is measured using various scales, including the Psoriasis Area and Severity Index (PASI), which considers surface area of plaques as well as symptom intensity. In a study of 2900 patients, two-thirds reported greater than 75% PASI improvement after 12 weeks of treatment, which increased to three-quarters after 24 weeks. Analysis of 545 patients with nail psoriasis revealed a greater than 45% improvement on the Nail Psoriasis Index plus a decrease in the number of psoriatic nails at 24 weeks with continued improvement at 52 weeks.[16] Nearly 50% of patients with psoriatic arthritis reported significant symptom reduction at 24 weeks using ustekinumab as compared with methotrexate and TNFα inhibitors.[17] Long-term data suggest ustekinumab is well tolerated and has no serious risks, but the cost of treatment leads some patients to discontinue therapy.[18]

Tumor Necrosis Factor Alpha Inhibitors

The mechanism of psoriasis involves activated T cells traveling to the epidermis and dermis and secreting type I cytokines to cause both proliferation and decreased maturation of keratinocytes.[19] An important factor in this pathologic process is the presence of the proinflammatory cytokine TNFα. Studies have shown increased levels of TNFα within the mast cells associated with psoriasiform lesions.[19] A treatment model has been used in studies to determine a mechanism of action for reducing the proinflammatory effects of TNFα in psoriasis. It is founded on 4 concepts: reduction of pathogenic T cells, inhibition of T cell activation, immune deviation of Th1 cells, and blockage of inflammatory cytokine activity.[20] Based on this model, biological therapy using TNFα inhibitors aims to antagonize the pathologic effects of the TNFα without causing organ toxicity associated with other systemic therapies.

Infliximab is a chimeric immunoglobulin monoclonal antibody that binds circulating TNFα and prevents it from activating respective receptors. Along with the treatment of psoriasis, infliximab is indicated for moderate-to-severe rheumatoid arthritis, Crohn disease, and unresponsive fistulating disease.[19] The drug is administered by intravenous infusion over a period of 2 hours. In addition to decreasing serum levels, it reduces cell infiltration, which leads to less keratinocyte proliferation.[19] Another widely used TNFα inhibitor is etanercept, a recombinant TNFα receptor fusion protein. Etanercept therapy seeks to neutralize the proinflammatory effects of TNFα and lymphotoxin-α. It is injected subcutaneously twice a week for the treatment of psoriasis and psoriatic arthritis. Overall, TNFα inhibitors are efficacious therapies that do not cause systemic toxicities as methotrexate.[19] The most common adverse effect for drugs in this class are infusion or injection site reactions.[21] Despite their therapeutic potential, TNFα inhibitors are limited by the pharmacoeconomics behind their production.[22] Biologics are specific molecules that cannot be precisely replicated; therefore, biosimilar molecules cannot be considered generic and would require clinical testing to determine efficacy.[20]

Interleukin-17 Inhibitors

New studies have investigated the use of biologics to target IL-17 in the treatment of moderate-to-severe psoriasis. They demonstrate that Th17 cells, in conjunction with Th1 and Th22 cells, infiltrate psoriatic plaques and secrete inflammatory mediators such as IL-17, TNFα, and IL-22 involved in the pathogenesis of psoriasis.[23,24] The prototype cytokine produced by Th17 cells is IL-17A, one member of the family of 6 IL-17 ligands ranging from A to F. These ligands combine in various combinations as homodimers, ultimately binding to 5 specific receptors (IL-17RA) to exert their activity.[25] Because of the involvement of IL-17 in the inflammatory cycle, 3 biologics are being studied for their targeted approach to psoriasis treatment: brodalumab, secukinumab, and ixekizumab. Each is approved for use in moderate-to-severe psoriasis, although secukinumab is also used for psoriatic arthritis.

Brodalumab is a human monoclonal antibody that binds IL-17RA, preventing its activation via IL-17A, IL-17F, and other isoforms. Targeting IL-17RA was previously shown to reverse psoriatic gene expression in the short term.[26] Two competing phase III clinical trials, AMAGINE-1 and AMAGINE-2, compared the efficacy of brodalumab to placebo and ustekinumab.[27] After 12 weeks, the highest number of patients exhibiting 75% to 100% improvement on the PASI were those receiving brodalumab. Despite significantly better outcomes, brodalumab was associated with side effects including nasopharyngitis, headache, upper respiratory tract infections, and even death due to stroke, cardiac arrest, and suicide. As a result, brodalumab was approved in the United States with a black box warning for suicide and risk management prevention.

Secukinumab, a fully human IgG4 monoclonal antibody, targets the IL-17A ligand and neutralizes its action on receptors. In total, there have been 7 phase III clinical trials that substantiate the validity of using secukinumab for the treatment of psoriasis and psoriatic arthritis.[28,29] In the most recent trials, it was shown to be effective in patients who previously did not respond well to nonsteroidal antiinflammatory drugs, disease-modifying antirheumatic drugs (DMARDs), and/or TNFα inhibitor therapy. Secukinumab significantly reduced the signs and symptoms of psoriatic arthritis, inhibited progression of the disease radiographically, and greatly improved overall quality of life. Furthermore, secukinumab was shown to outperform etanercept.[30] Side effects were mild and included nasopharyngitis, headache, upper respiratory tract infection, and diarrhea.[29,30]

Ixekizumab is another human monoclonal antibody that binds the IL-17A ligand, antagonizing its proinflammatory action.[31] The US Food and Drug Administration approved ixekizumab for the treatment of moderate-to-severe psoriasis based on the results of several phase III clinical trials. SPIRIT-P1 showed improved skin and joint manifestations as well as improved quality of life in patients with psoriatic arthritis that was previously unresponsive to DMARDs.[32] Similar results are out in SPIRIT-P2, a larger study that also included patients whose disease had not responded well to TNFα inhibitors.[33] Finally, the 3 most recents trials, UNCOVER-1, -2 and -3, demonstrated that patients taking ixekizumab for 12 weeks had better outcomes than those using etanercept with respect to psoriasis and psoriatic arthritis.[34] Supplemental data after 60 weeks support these findings. Treatment with ixekizumab most resulted in candidal infections, neutropenia, and inflammatory bowel disease.

SUMMARY

Psoriasis is a chronic autoimmune disease that causes systemic inflammation, which usually presents as skin lesions. Besides physical pain and disability, patients suffer emotional stress from its effect on their visual appearance. The challenges in achieving remission of moderate-to-severe psoriasis have sparked research into novel treatment options. Most recently, biologics have emerged as effective pharmacotherapeutic agents in the treatment of psoriasis (skin and nails) and psoriatic arthritis following the failure of first-line treatments. Classes of biologics such as IL-23 inhibitors, IL-12/23 inhibitors, TNFα inhibitors, and IL-17 inhibitors have yielded promising results in the alleviation of symptoms by inhibiting cytokines crucial in the recruitment of immune cells. Clinical trials clearly show these agents improve patient symptoms, but larger studies are needed to determine their prolonged efficacy and side-effect profile to draw definitive conclusions regarding their place as standard treatments for moderate-to-severe psoriasis. Further research is warranted to reduce the high cost of many biologics and make them more economically viable options for all patients. Nonetheless, encouraging progress has been made in developing biological agents that improve the quality of life of patients suffering from this debilitating condition, especially on the lower extremity.

CLINICS CARE POINTS

- Ustekinumab is a human immunoglobulin G (IgG) 1 kappa monoclonal antibody that binds the p40 subunit found in IL-12 and IL-23.
- Infliximab is a chimeric immunoglobulin monoclonal antibody that binds circulating TNFa and prevents it from activating respective receptors. Along with the treatment of psoriasis, infliximab is also indicated for moderate-to-severe rheumatoid arthritis.
- Ixekizumab is another human monoclonal antibody that binds the IL-17A ligand, antagonizing its proinflammatory action which has been approved for the treatment of moderate-to-severe psoriasis.

REFERENCES

1. Torre KM, Payette MJ. Combination biologic therapy for the treatment of palmoplantar pustulosis. J Am Acad Dermatol 2017;3(3):240–2.
2. Psoriasis [Internet]. Rosemont, IL: American Academy of Dermatology (AAD); 2018. Available from: https://www.aad.org/public/diseases/scaly-skin/psoriasis#symptoms. Accessed April 9, 2018.
3. Psoriasis - symptoms and causes. Scottsdale, AZ: Mayo Foundation for Medical Education and Research (MFMER); 1998-2018. Available from: https://www.mayoclinic.org/diseases-conditions/psoriasis/symptoms-causes/syc-20355840. Accessed April 11, 2018.
4. The Psoriatic Foot. St. Albans, Hertfordshire, UK: Psoriasis and Psoriatic Arthritis Alliance (PAPAA); 1993-2018. Available from: http://www.papaa.org/further-information/pustular-psoriasis. Accessed April 7, 2018.
5. Miceli A, Schmieder GJ. Palmoplantar Psoriasis. [Updated 2020 Aug 15]. In: StatPearls [Internet]. Treasure Island (FL): StatPearls Publishing; 2021. Available at: https://www.ncbi.nlm.nih.gov/books/NBK448142/.

6. Moderate to severe psoriasis: biologic drugs. Portland, OR: National Psoriasis Foundation/USA; 1996-2018. Available from: https://www.psoriasis.org/about-psoriasis/treatments/biologics. Accessed April 6, 2018.

7. Di Cesare A, Di Meglio P, Nestle FO. The IL-23/Th17 axis in the immunopathogenesis of psoriasis. J Invest Dermatol 2009;129(6):1339–50.

8. Tonel G, Conrad C, Laggner U, et al. Cutting edge: a critical functional role for IL-23 in psoriasis. J Immunol 2010;185(10):5688–91.

9. Sofen H, Smith S, Matheson RT, et al. Guselkumab (an IL-23–specific mAb) demonstrates clinical and molecular response in patients with moderate-to-severe psoriasis. J Allergy Clin Immunol 2014;133(4):1032–40.

10. Reich K, Armstrong AW, Foley P, et al. Efficacy and safety of guselkumab, an anti-interleukin-23 monoclonal antibody, compared with adalimumab for the treatment of patients with moderate to severe psoriasis with randomized withdrawal and re-treatment: results from the phase III, double-blind, placebo- and active comparator–controlled VOYAGE 2 trial. J Am Acad Dermatol 2017;76(3):418–31.

11. Benson J, Peritt D, Scallon B, et al. Discovery and mechanism of ustekinumab. MAbs 2011;3(6):535–45.

12. Yielding N, Szepary P, Brodmerkel C, et al. Development of the IL-12/23 antagonist ustekinumab in psoriasis: past, present, and future perspectives. Ann N Y Acad Sci 2011;1222:30–9.

13. Bartlett BL, Moody MN, Tyring SK. IL-12/IL-23 inhibitors: the advantages and disadvantages of this novel approach for the treatment of psoriasis. Skin Therapy Lett 2008;13(8):1–4.

14. Thaci D, Blauvelt A, Reich K, et al. Secukinumab is superior to ustekinumab in clearing skin of subjects with moderate to severe plaque psoriasis: CLEAR, a randomized controlled trial. J Am Acad Dermatol 2015;73(3):400–9.

15. Duvallet E, Semerano L, Assier E, et al. Interleukin-23: a key cytokine in inflammatory diseases. Ann Med 2011;43(7):503–11.

16. Rich P, Bourcier M, Sofen H, et al. Ustekinumab improves nail disease in patients with moderate-to-severe psoriasis: results from Phoenix 1. Br J Dermatol 2013; 170(2):398–407.

17. Ritchlin C, Rahman P, Kavanaugh A, et al. Efficacy and safety of the anti-IL-12/23 p40 monoclonal antibody, ustekinumab, in patients with active psoriatic arthritis despite conventional non-biological and biological anti-tumour necrosis factor therapy: 6-month and 1-year results of the phase 3, multicentre, double-blind, placebo-controlled, randomised PSUMMIT 2 trial. Ann Rheum Dis 2014;73: 990–9.

18. Choi CW, Choi JY, Kim BR, et al. Economic burden can be the major determining factor resulting in short-term intermittent and repetitive ustekinumab treatment for moderate-to-severe psoriasis. Ann Dermatol 2018;30(2):179–85.

19. Kirby B, Tobin A. TNF- α in the treatment of psoriasis and psoriatic arthritis. BioDrugs 2005;19(1):47–57.

20. Weinberg JM. Biologic therapy for psoriasis: an overview of infliximab, etanercept, adalimumab, efalizumab, and alefacept. Treat Psoriasis 2003;25(10): 141–58.

21. Khurana A, Pandhi D, Sehgal VN. Biologics in dermatology: adverse effects. Int J Dermatol 2015;54(12):1442–60.

22. Kimball AB, Porter ML. Pharmacoeconomics of systemic and biologic therapy in dermatology. Biol Systemic Agents Dermatol 2018;83–91.

23. Nestle FO, Kaplan DH, Barker J, et al. Psoriasis. N Engl J Med 2009;361(5): 496–509.

24. Nestle FO, Di Meglio P, Qin JZ, et al. Skin immune sentinels in health and disease. Nat Rev Immunol 2009;9(10):679–91.
25. Gaffen SL. Recent advances in the IL-17 cytokine family. Curr Opin Immunol 2011;23(5):613–9.
26. Russell CB, Rand H, Bigler J, et al. Gene expression profiles normalized in psoriatic skin by treatment with brodalumab, a human anti-IL-17 receptor monoclonal antibody. J Immunol 2014;192:3828–36.
27. Lebwohl M, Strober B, Menter A, et al. Phase 3 studies comparing brodalumab with ustekinumab in psoriasis. N Engl J Med 2015;373:1318–28.
28. Mease PJ, McInnes IB, Kirkham B, et al. Secukinumab inhibition of interleukin-17A in patients with psoriatic arthritis. N Engl J Med 2015;373(14):1329–39.
29. McInnes IB, Mease PJ, Kirkham B, et al. Secukinumab, a human anti-interleukin-17A monoclonal antibody, in patients with psoriatic arthritis (FUTURE 2): a randomised, double-blind, placebo-controlled, phase 3 trial. Lancet 2015;386: 1137–46.
30. Langley RG, Elewski BE, Lebwohl M, et al. Secukinumab in plaque psoriasis–results of two phase 3 trials. N Engl J Med 2014;371(4):326–38.
31. Ren V, Dao H. Potential role of ixekizumab in the treatment of moderate-to-severe plaque psoriasis. Clin Cosmet Investig Dermatol 2013;6:75–80.
32. Van Der Heijde D, Gladman DD, Kishimoto M, et al. Efficacy and safety of ixekizumab in patients with active psoriatic arthritis: 52-week results from a phase III study (SPIRIT-P1). J Rheumatol 2018;45:3.
33. Nach P, Kirkham B, Okada M, et al. Ixekizumab for the treatment of patients with active psoriatic arthritis and an inadequate response to tumour necrosis factor inhibitors: results from the 24-week randomised, double-blind, placebo-controlled period of the SPIRIT-P2 phase 3 trial. Lancet 2017;389(10086):2317–27.
34. Gordon KB, Blauvelt A, Papp KA, et al. Phase 3 trials of ixekizumab in moderate-to-severe plaque psoriasis. N Engl J Med 2016;375:334–56.

Shoe Dermatitis

Victoria Adeniran, DPM, Asher Cherian, DPM, Jin O. Cho, DPM,
Ciesco Febrian, DPM, Eui T. Kim, DPM, Tymoteusz Siwy, DPM,
Tracey C. Vlahovic, DPM*

KEYWORDS

- Shoe dermatitis • Allergic contact dermatitis • Irritant contact dermatitis

KEY POINTS

- Allergic contact dermatitis (ACD) caused by exposure to footwear may occur from a variety of agents found in any part of the shoe. Also known as shoe dermatitis, the most common allergens are from leather, rubber, and adhesives.
- A patch test can distinguish ACD from ICD, which directs the source of the reaction and patient treatment course.
- Both conservative and pharmacologic treatments, such as shoegear changes, barrier creams, and topical corticosteroids are mainstays of contact dermatitis therapy.

INTRODUCTION

Allergic contact dermatitis (ACD) caused by exposure to footwear may occur from a variety of agents found in any part of the shoe. Also known as shoe dermatitis, the most common allergens are from leather, rubber, and adhesives.[1–5] Socks must also not be overlooked as a source of allergens because reports exist of patients reacting to rubbers and dyes in socks.[3] Shoe dermatitis presents as both acute and chronic phases. Pruritus and lesion severity can be used as a differentiating marker for mimickers, including tinea pedis and lichen planus.[2,6] The impact of shoe dermatitis is not limited to particular races or cultures. It is important to identify the offending agent or agents to help patients avoid further exposure, a key initial step in the treatment of both phases of ACD.[1–5,7–11] If conservative treatments are not effective, pharmacologic agents are also available to ease the burden of the skin disease.[2,8,12]

Dermatitis is an interchangeable term with eczema and represents a blanket term that is not specific. A form of dermatitis, contact dermatitis (CD) is a broad term for the inflammatory skin reaction due to direct contact with a noxious agent in the environment. CD includes both nonimmunologic irritant contact dermatitis (ICD) and the immunologically mediated ACD.[2,6]

Conflict of Interest: None of the authors have any financial interests to disclose for this article.
Temple University School of Podiatric Medicine, 148 North 8th Street, Philadelphia, PA 19107, USA
* Corresponding author.
E-mail address: traceyv@temple.edu

ICD is thought to have multiple interlinked pathways involved and is the most common of occupational CD cases. ICD can be caused by physical, mechanical, or chemical causes and results from the direct contact with irritants and damage to the skin. ICD is also known to be the most common cause of hand eczema.[2,6]

ACD is caused by a variety of different allergens, and the causative allergens vary with the population considered. Among the variety of possible allergens, top contributing allergens are often included in shoe materials, such as rubber, dye, and fragrances. Studies have shown that throughout the history of shoe dermatitis, allergens with the highest number of positive patch test results are potassium dichromate, mercapto mix, thiuram mix, and fragrance mix.[1,13] One study showed that among the British Contact Dermatitis Society Standard series, potassium dichromate was found to be the most prevalent cause of CD with the highest number of populations reacting to patch test, followed by neomycin, mercapto mix, and thiuram mix, in decreasing order.[14]

With new shoe products on the market, several new allergens have been found to cause ACD. Dimethyl-thiocarbamylbenzothiazole sulfide (DMTBS) is a material used in the new canvas "Sperry Top-Sider" model. The extracts of the shoe were analyzed and patch tested with varying degrees of dilution and showed positive results with symptoms increasing in severity as the concentration of DMTBS increased.[15]

Shoe refreshers have also been proved to be a new allergen causing shoe dermatitis. Positive patch test results were shown with diluted shoe refreshers.[16] In a patch test study using a sample of shin pad products, acetophenone azine showed positive results in both pediatric and adult populations.[17]

Other common contributory allergens of shoe dermatitis in India include leather and leather-related chemicals, cobalt chloride, paraphenylenediamine, epoxy resin, nickel sulfate, colophony, p-tert-butyl-formaldehyde resin, and formaldehyde.[18]

PRESENTATION

Pathologic presentation of ICD and ACD may be difficult to differentiate, because both present a spongiotic reaction pattern and epidermal edema. Necrosis of keratinocytes is linked with ICD, whereas vesiculation with mild exocytosis and presence of eosinophils is reflective of the immunologic nature of ACD. The common office presentation of a patient with dermatitis is a red and scaly rash. The patient interview best guides the physician to believe that it is a skin reaction to something that he or she has been exposed to.[19]

In general, CD has acute, subacute, and chronic phases. The acute phase is characterized by pruritus with an erythematous scaling and oozing skin rash with or without vesicles. The subacute form has a milder presentation of the same symptoms: less erythematous, pruritic, scaling, and fissured skin rash. The 2 types of CD are nonimmunologic ICD and immunologic ACD. Unlike ICD, the course of ACD involves previous exposure to an offending agent causing a sensitization process. In ACD, the sensitization process allows one or more exposures to the allergen before presenting as an eczematous skin reaction.[20] Spreading of the ACD reaction can occur by scratching the affected site and subsequently scratching another area of the body. Immunologic ACD also has acute, subacute, and chronic phases. ACD usually presents with bilateral, symmetric eczematous lesions on the dorsum of the foot while sparing the interdigital space.[2] The chronic form of the ACD can cause the skin to become lichenified, fissured, or pigmented.

Shoe ACD occurs in 1.5% to 24% of patch-tested patients.[1,21] Shoe dermatitis has a predilection for men because they wear tight or ill-fitting footwear for long periods, whereas women develop it due to variation in footwear.[20,22] Shoe ACD is characterized by the presence of erythema, papules, vesicles, oozing, scaling, and crusting at the site of contact. Acral skin can facilitate the transfer of allergens to other parts of the body, therefore these signs can be present anywhere on the body or foot but are most common on the dorsum of the foot.[2,22]

PATHOPHYSIOLOGY AND MECHANISMS OF CONTACT DERMATITIS
Irritant Contact Dermatitis

Direct disruption of the barrier function of the stratum corneum by chemicals and physical agents elicits the nonimmunologic cutaneous ICD response. The stratum corneum provides a 2-way checkpoint to prevent transepidermal water loss as well as an entry barrier of irritants or allergens. Corneocytes with a complex layer of intercellular lipids, ceramides, cholesterol, and free fatty acids make up the stratum corneum. The corneocytes also produce natural moisturizing factor, a complex layer of lipids that helps to retain moisture.[6,23,24]

The integrity of the stratum corneum also depends on its slightly acidic environment. The integrity can be imbalanced by a constant barrage of irritants, which results in the impairment of skin's ability to regenerate. Hand washing causes the pH to become more alkaline; however, a more acidic pH environment of the stratum corneum will help to create a bactericidal environment. Apart from altering pH, frequent washing with soaps and detergents also disrupts the lipid bilayer and the natural moisturizing factor of the skin.

Acute skin tissue disruptions increase skin permeability and transepidermal water loss. The injury induces the release of cytokines and tumor necrosis factor α from keratinocytes, leading to release of further proinflammatory chemokines, attracting mononuclear and polymorphonuclear cells at the site of injury. Resolution of the inflammatory process occurs with induction of anti-inflammatory cytokines simultaneously released from the keratinocytes.

ICD can develop with enough repeated exposure to an irritant; however, prior sensitization is not required. Atopic dermatitis, linked to a null mutation in the filaggrin gene, is associated with persistent fissured skin and increased nickel sensitization, and as a result susceptibility to ICD. Some patients may develop tolerance to repeated exposure of irritants through changes in lipid composition, permeability of skin, and inflammatory mediators inducing the hardening phenomenon.[2,24]

Allergic Contact Dermatitis

ACD is a type IV hypersensitivity, a T-cell-mediated delayed response. ACD develops more slowly because antigen-specific effector T cells require induced synthesis of effector molecules. Contact hypersensitivity antigens typically are highly reactive small molecules that can penetrate skin and are induced by itching and scratching. Antigens include small metal ions nickel and chromate, as well as haptens. Chemicals that are electrophilic, including compounds with polarized bond, unsaturated compounds, or cations, including nickel and chromate, react to form haptens that lead to skin sensitization.[23] Haptens react with self-proteins to form a protein-hapten complex, which gets processed to hapten-peptide complexes by Langerhans cells, which then bind to major histocompatibility complex to be presented to T cells as foreign antigens. A local epidermal reaction then occurs, which includes erythema, cellular infiltrate, vesiculation, and intraepidermal abscess. This process is divided into the sensitization and elicitation phases.[2,6,23,25]

The sensitization phase of the ACD hypersensitivity response process begins with the cutaneous Langerhans cells taking up and processing the antigen. The Langerhans cells then migrate to the regional lymph nodes where they activate T cells, which then induce the production of memory T cells. The T cells then migrate to the site of effect in the dermis. Sensitization is followed by elicitation in which further exposure to the sensitizing chemical leads to presentation to memory T cells in the dermis, leading to activation and further recruitment of specific T cells. Activation and recruitment occurs with the release of T cell cytokines such as interferon-gamma and interleukin-17 stimulating keratinocytes of the epidermis to release cytokines; this leads to increased inflammatory response with an increased migration and maturation monocytes into the lesion, also leading to attraction of more T cells to the site.[2,6,23,25]

EPIDEMIOLOGY

Shoe dermatitis affects multiple ethnicities and geographic regions. In a study conducted by the North American Contact Dermatitis Group, 19,457 patients were tested with 45 allergens in 13 centers in North America, including major allergens of shoe dermatitis. The study found that 92.9% (17,803) were Caucasians and 7.1% (1360) were African Americans. The overall patch test positive rates were similar for most allergens between the 2 groups. However, African American patients reacted more frequently to shoe allergens. The US African American population had higher allergic reaction rates to bacitracin/neomycin, mercaptobenzothiazole (rubber), thiuram, and mercapto mix. However, the Caucasian population had a higher allergic reaction rate to dyes/fragrances and formaldehyde. The causes of these differences are unknown.[26,27]

According to a study done by the Contact and Occupational Dermatoses Forum of India among a total of 640 patch-tested patients, the proportion of shoe dermatitis was 24.22% or 155 patients. There were more females, 61.93% or 96 patients, and male patients comprised only 38.06% or 59 patients. Patient age distribution was from 8 to 75 years, showing that anyone who wears shoes is potentially exposed to risk of shoe dermatitis. The most prevalently involved age group was the fifth decade, 24.52% or 38 patients. The most prevalently involved occupation group was housewives, comprising 42.58% or 66 patients.[18]

DIFFERENTIAL DIAGNOSES

Hallmark signs of dermatitis include calor, rubor, tumor, and pruritus. Pruritus can be used a differentiating marker for other conditions that mimic dermatitis in visual presentation.[2,6] A red and scaly rash, the appearance of foot CD, may be due to several diseases, including tinea pedis, psoriasis, or lichen planus. Other possibilities include mechanical irritant dermatitis, juvenile plantar dermatosis, and atopic eczema.[28] However, patient history, physical examination, and clinical appearance may eliminate many of the possibilities. In cases wherein some differentials are eliminated but the disease source cannot be discerned, a patch test will distinguish ACD from ICD.[20,29]

Atopic dermatitis, dyshidrotic eczema, and palmoplantar psoriasis are the differential diagnoses of CD, but these can be diagnosed with skin biopsy. Unlike CD, atopic dermatitis is more widespread, however, and distributes along flexor surfaces. Dyshidrotic eczema also presents with deep-seated, tapiocalike vesicles and occurs on the hands more frequently than the feet. Palmoplantar psoriasis tends to present as localized plaques and pustules rather than a generalized rash.[28]

Furthermore, latex allergy, scabies, and tinea pedis may present like CD, but can be diagnosed with allergy testing, skin scraping, and potassium hydroxide testing, respectively. Latex allergy may also present with a systemic reaction. Scabies presents with burrows that are typically distributed in the groin, axilla, waist, and hands in addition to the feet. Moreover, tinea pedis usually occurs between the toes rather than on the dorsum of the foot.[28]

TREATMENTS FOR SHOE DERMATITIS
Elimination of Allergens/Irritants and Creating Physical Barriers

The approach in treating ACD and ICD is to first identify the causative agent followed by the avoidance of the offending allergen and irritant in the patient's environment. In addition to obtaining a thorough patient history, patch testing is recommended to determine the offending agent or agents and better direct treatment and patient education.[1–11] Suitable replacement for shoes and socks lacking the offending compounds may be readily available or may require custom manufacturing. Freeman[1] report that by replacing leather inner soles with cork inner soles and wearing moccasin-style footwear free of rubber adhesives, patients reported improvements in shoe dermatitis symptoms. When ACD is caused by chromium salts, compounds commonly used in leather processing tanning and dyeing, it is best to direct patients to purchase shoes or boots made from chromium-free leather or alternative materials.[3,5] In cases in which an alternative shoe style cannot be implemented for practical or safety reasons patients may apply a double layer of socks to increase the barrier between dorsal and plantar foot skin, and offending materials and adhesives contained in shoes. Patients should be advised that double socking may result in requiring shoes that are a half size larger.[1,3] High-quality leather shoes containing chromium compounds may be used but may need to be discarded and replaced after a few months of use. Hyperhidrosis may shorten the useable lifespan of such shoes because increased sweating may precipitate chromate lixiviating from the leather.[3,5]

Special fabrics are available to palliate the symptoms of ACD and ICD. Cotton is a possible cause of mild irritation and exacerbation of ICD. Ricci and colleagues[30] compared the use of topical moisturizers with that of woven silk fabric (Microair Derma-Silk by Alpretec) in pediatric patients, with topical moisturizer and cotton fabric being used as control. Statistically significant improvement was noted in patients using woven silk garments.[30] A recent study by Corazza and colleagues[9] examined another Microair multilayer material used in socks and undergarments engineered by Alpretec designed to increase perspirability and block allergens and irritants. This material is a microporous membrane core interposed between polyester microfiber piqué. Most participants reported a reduction in itch (66%), pain reduction (77%), and improvement in their ability to walk without pain (100%) after 8 weeks of exclusively wearing Microair barrier socks. It should be noted that the sample size of this study was small and did not include a control group. Furthermore, 66% of the participants noted difficulties in wearing Microair socks daily due to discomfort and esthetic reasons.[3,9]

Pharmacologic Treatment

Emollients and humectants such as urea and glycerol are some of the most common therapeutics prescribed for ACD and ICD to maintain skin hydration by trapping water in the epidermis. Maintaining skin hydration is crucial in protecting and restoring skin integrity, thus maintaining the patient's natural protective barrier. Anti-inflammatory agents, antipruritic agents, and epithelium growth-promoting agents may also be included in emollient or humectant preparations.[2,31,32] Emollient preparations may contain vehicles such as propylene glycol that can trigger or exacerbate ICD, requiring close patient monitoring.[2,3]

Barrier creams are sometimes included in ACD and ICD prophylaxis. The proposed mechanism is to establish a physical barrier between the epidermis and the outside world. Lipophilic preparations should offer protection against lipophobic irritants and allergens, and lipophobic preparations should offer protection against lipophilic irritants and allergens.[12,32,33] Some preparations contain chelating agents such as clioquinol to decrease transdermal absorption of metals such as zinc and nickel. The benefits of barrier creams have been debated for a long time, and there is no strong consensus pertaining to their efficacy, in part due to the large number of active compounds and vehicle combinations.[2,3,7,12,33] Brendt and colleagues[34] suggest that the active ingredients in protective creams are no more effective as skin protectants than preparation vehicle alone (no statistically significant difference found). The investigators attribute this to glycerin (vehicle) being a good moisturizer allowing skin rehydration and regeneration.

Topical corticosteroids are an important mainstay of ACD management. Corticosteroid-mediated inhibition of a localized immune response via inhibition of T cell activation and leukocyte migration is a crucial process in arresting the hypersensitivity reaction causing ACD. A short-term course of a topical corticosteroid may be sufficient in the treatment of a patient with ACD.[2,3,8,35] It is important to consider a paradoxic side effect of topical corticosteroid use: a short-term application of a potent corticosteroid such as clobetasol or betamethasone may result in epidermal thinning and compromise of the skin barrier.[2,8] The utility of topical corticosteroids in the treatment of ICD is limited.[8]

Calcineurin inhibitors (pimecrolimus and tacrolimus) are immunosuppressant drugs causing the upstream inhibition of activation of the NFAT transcription factor, resulting in decreased production of proinflammatory cytokines.[8,36] In addition, pimecrolimus inhibits cytokine production in mast cells.[36] Tacrolimus and pimecrolimus are both effective topical agents for the treatment of ACD. Topical pimecrolimus is more selective to the skin due to 20-fold greater lipophilicity compared with tacrolimus, but it is also 3-fold less potent than topical tacrolimus.[8,36] Cyclosporine is an oral calcineurin inhibitor effective against severe ACD and is used in patients who do not respond to topical corticosteroid therapy. Cyclosporine administration should be concomitant with patient monitoring for hypertension and renal dysfunction, potentially serious side effects of cyclosporine.[2,37] Cyclosporine has limited capability to pass through the epidermis, hindering its use as a topical agent.[8]

Phototherapy using UV-B and topical psoralen with UV-A (PUVA) light exposure is ordinarily performed in patients who have failed previous courses of treatment or have refractory ACD. The therapeutic property of phototherapy is attributed to the immunosuppressive properties of UV light.[2,8] Both PUVA and UV-B therapies yield excellent results in treating ACD and ICD, with no statistically significant differences in outcomes between treatments with PUVA or UV-B. PUVA may produce more phototoxic side effects, suggesting that UV-B phototherapy should be attempted first before progressing to PUVA. However, both modalities experienced high relapse rates within months of discontinuing therapy, indicating a need for continued maintenance treatment to prevent ACD or ICD recurrence.[8]

SUMMARY

Although there are many allergen and irritant causes of shoe dermatitis, and many other diseases that resemble it, proper diagnosis and treatment is possible. The importance of a thorough patient history and physical examination cannot be underestimated. Furthermore, a patch test can distinguish ACD from ICD, which directs the source of the reaction and patient treatment course. Both conservative and pharmacologic treatments, such as shoegear changes, barrier creams, and topical corticosteroids may lead to CD resolution. There is still room for discovery of the reasons behind the apparent higher prevalence of CD in African Americans compared with Caucasians, behind epidemiology differences in other nations, and regarding overcoming limitations of current pharmacologic treatments.

CLINICS CARE POINTS

- Atopic dermatitis, dyshidrotic eczema, and palmoplantar psoriasis are the differential diagnoses of contact dermatitis, but these can be diagnosed with skin biopsy.

- ACD is caused by a variety of different allergens, and the causative allergens vary. Among the variety of possible allergens, top allergens are often included in shoe materials, such as rubber, dye, and fragrances.

- Emollients and humectants such as urea and glycerol are some of the most common therapeutics prescribed for ACD and ICD to maintain skin hydration by trapping water in the epidermis. Maintaining skin hydration is crucial in protecting and restoring skin integrity, thus maintaining the patient's natural protective barrier.

REFERENCES

1. Freeman S. Shoe dermatitis. Contact Dermatitis 1997;36:247–51.
2. Bangash HK, Petronic-Rosic V. Acral manifestations of contact dermatitis. Clin Dermatol 2017;35:9–18.
3. Matthys E, Zahir A, Ehrlich A. Shoe allergic contact dermatitis. Am Contact Dermatitis Soc 2014;25:163.
4. Lecamwasam K, Latheef F, Walker B, et al. Contact allergy to reactive dyes in footwear. Contact Dermatitis 2017;76:370.
5. Landeck L, Uter W, John SW. Patch test characteristics of patients referred for suspected contact allergy of the feet – retrospective 10-year cross-sectional study of the IVDK data. Contact Dermatitis 2012;66:271.
6. Vlahovic TC, Schleicher SM. Skin disease of the lower extremities: a photographic guide. Malvern (PA): HMP Communications; 2012.
7. Al-Otaibi ST, Alqahtani HAM. Management of contact dermatitis. J Dermatol Dermatol Surg 2015;19:86.
8. Cohen DE, Heidary N. Treatment of irritant and allergic contact dermatitis. Dermatol Ther 2004;17:334.
9. Corazza M, Baldo F, Ricci M, et al. Efficacy of new barrier socks in the treatment of foot allergic contact dermatitis. Acta Derm Venereol 2011;91:68.
10. Ibler KS, Jemec GBE, Diepgen TL, et al. Skin care education and individual counseling versus treatment as usual in healthcare workers with hand eczema: randomized clinical trial. BMJ 2012;345:1.
11. Jacob SE, Burk CJ, Connelly EA. Patch testing: another steroid-sparing agent to consider in children. Pediatr Dermatol 2008;25:81.
12. Alvarez MS, Brown LH, Brancaccio RR. Are barrier creams actually effective? Curr Allergy Asthma Rep 2001;1:337.
13. Cockayne S, Shah M, Messenger A, et al. Foot dermatitis in children: causative allergens and follow-up. Contact Dermatitis 1998;38:203–6.
14. Holden CR, Gawkrodger DJ. 10 years' experience of patch testing with a shoe series in 230 patients: which allergens are important? Contact Dermatitis 2005;53:37–9.
15. Hulstaert E, Bergendorff O, Persson C, et al. Contact dermatitis caused by a new rubber compound detected in canvas shoes. Contact Dermatitis 2018;78:12–7.
16. Mowitz M, Ponten A. Foot dermatitis caused by didecyldimethylammonium chloride in an shoe refresher spray. Contact Dermatitis 2015;73:364–80.
17. Charlotte D, Bergendorff O, Raison-Peyron N, et al. Acetophenone azine: a new shoe allergen causing severe foot dermatitis. Contact Dermatitis 2017;77:406–29.

18. Chowdhuri S, Ghosh S. Epidemio-allergological study in 155 cases of footwear dermatitis. Indian J Dermatol Venereol Leprol 2007;73:319–22.
19. Wilkinson M, Orton D. Allergic contact dermatitis. In: Griffiths C, Barjer J, Bleiker T, et al, editors. Rook's textbook of dermatology. 9th edition. Indianapolis (IN): John Wiley & Sons; 2016. p. 128.4.
20. Matthys E1, Zahir A, Ehrlich A. Shoe allergic contact dermatitis. Dermatitis 2014; 25(4):163–71.
21. Saha M, Srinivas CR, Shenoy SD, et al. Footwear dermatitis. Contact Dermatitis 1993;28(5):260–4.
22. Rani Z, Hussain I, Haroon TS. Common allergens in shoe dermatitis: our experience in Lahore, Pakistan. Int J Dermatol 2003;42(8):605–7.
23. Divkovic M, Pease CK, Gerberick GF, et al. Hapten-protein binding: from theory to practical application in the in vitro prediction of skin sensitization. Contact Dermatitis 2005;53(4):189–200.
24. Tan C-H, Rasool S, Johnston GA. Contact dermatitis: allergic and irritant. Clin Dermatol 2014;32(1):116–24.
25. Janeway CA Jr, Travers P, Walport M, et al. Immunobiology: the immune system in health and disease. 5th edition. New York: Garland Science; 2001. Available at: https://www.ncbi.nlm.nih.gov/books/NBK10757/.
26. Deleo VA, Alexis A, Warshaw EM, Sasseville Denis. The association of race/ethnicity and patch test results: North American contact dermatitis group, 1998-2006. Dermatitis 2016;27(No. 5):288–92.
27. Onder M, Atahan AC, Bassoy B. Foot dermatitis from the shoes. Int J Dermatol 2004;43:565–7.
28. Usatine RP, Riojas M. Diagnosis and management of contact dermatitis. Am Fam Physician 2010;82:249–55.
29. Lee HY, Stieger M, Yawalkar N, et al. Cytokines and chemokines in irritant contact dermatitis. Mediators Inflamm 2013;2013:916497.
30. Ricci G, Patrizi A, Bendandi B, et al. Clinical effectiveness of a silk fabric in the treatment of atopic dermatitis. Br J Dermatol 2004;150:127.
31. Moncrieff G, Cork M, Lawton S, et al. Use of emollients in dry-skin conditions: consensus statement. Clin Exp Dermatol 2013;38:231.
32. Zhai H, Maibach HI. In: Chew AL, Maibach HI, editors. "Barrier creams and emollients" in irritant dermatitis. Berlin: Springer; 2006. p. 479.
33. Schliemann S, Petri M, Elsner P. Preventing irritant contact dermatitis with protective creams: influence of the application dose. Contact Dermatitis 2013;70:19.
34. Berndt U, Wigger-Alberti W, Gabard B, et al. Efficacy of a barrier cream and its vehicle as protective measures against occupational irritant contact dermatitis. Contact Dermatitis 2000;42:77.
35. Hachem JP, De Paepe K, Vanpée E, et al. Efficacy of topical corticosteroids in nickel-induced contact allergy. Clin Exp Dermatol 2002;27:47.
36. Gupta AK, Chow M. Pimecrolimus: a review. J Eur Acad Dermatol Venereol 2003; 17:493.
37. Flori L, Perotti R, Mazzatenta C, et al. Cyclosporin A in the treatment of severe allergic contact dermatitis. J Eur Acad Dermatol Venereol 1993;2:200.

Cutaneous Manifestations of the Diabetic Foot

Sam Gorelik, DPM, Alexander Leos, DPM, Amida Kuah, DPM, Salil Desai, DPM,
Ahmad Namous, DPM, Alexandru Onica, DPM, Tracey C. Vlahovic, DPM*

KEYWORDS

- Diabetes • Necrobiosis lipoidica • Onychomycosis • Psoriasis • Lichen planus
- Blisters • Dermopathy

KEY POINTS

- Skin conditions may be present in patients with diabetes before their formal diagnosis or after they have been diagnosed. Many conditions are related to blood glucose control.
- Skin manifestations may be seen in patients with type 1 or type 2 diabetes.
- Diabetic dermopathy is classically considered the most common skin condition.

INTRODUCTION

Diabetes mellitus (DM) is a highly prevalent disease in the United States. It is estimated that 30.3 million Americans (nearly 10% of the population) has DM and more than 30% of American adults are prediabetic.[1] DM involves the inability to break down glucose into a useable form of energy. Glucose accumulates within the bloodstream, which causes myriad unwanted consequences. DM is categorized into type 1 and type 2. Type 1 DM is due to autoimmune destruction of the pancreatic cells that produce insulin, a hormone required for glucose metabolism. In contrast, type 2 DM is due to normal or decreased insulin production with cellular resistance to the effects of insulin. Both types of DM present with symptoms such as increased thirst, frequent urination, and poor wound healing. We analyzed the cutaneous manifestations of both types of DM on the lower extremity.[1]

NECROBIOSIS LIPOIDICA

Necrobiosis lipoidica is a granulomatous disorder characterized by groups of papules that coalesce into well-circumscribed erythematous patches and plaques with yellow–brown centers. These lesions subsequently atrophy and tend to ulcerate, especially when subjected to trauma.[2–4] The patches and plaques, which form in the early stages of necrobiosis lipoidica, have decreased or no sensation.[5] The ulcers that form in the late stage of the disorder may become painful. Although the preulcerative lesions are

Conflict of Interest: None of the authors have any financial interests to disclose for this article.
Temple University School of Podiatric Medicine, 148 N 8th Street, Philadelphia, PA 19107, USA
* Corresponding author.
E-mail address: traceyv@temple.edu

generally asymptomatic, the complications of ulceration in necrobiosis lipoidica include secondary infection and possible progression to squamous cell carcinoma.[5] These lesions are most frequently located on the anterior surface of the leg, but may also occur on the dorsal surface of the foot or the heel (**Fig. 1**).

BULLOSIS DIABETICORUM

Bullosis diabeticorum involves the formation of diabetic bullae, which are intraepidermal or subepidermal sterile blisters ranging from a few millimeters and up to 5 cm in diameter.[2,4] A solitary blister or a group of blisters may develop spontaneously in patients suffering from long-standing diabetic peripheral neuropathy and usually resolve within 3 to 5 weeks, although recurrence is common. The major concern is infection of the blister.[4,5] These blisters are most frequently located on the anterior surface of the leg, the sides of the leg, or the dorsal surface of the foot.[6]

ERUPTIVE XANTHOMA

Eruptive xanthomas may present yellow papules with an erythematous base or as planar lesions that are yellow in color and form at major joints such as the elbows, knees, and gluteal region. These lesions may be seen in patients with type 2 diabetes.[7] Most cases of eruptive xanthomas are mistaken by the patient for an allergic reaction. Eruptive xanthomas typically form owing to decreased activity of lipoprotein lipase and increased levels of triglycerides. Circulating lipids aggregate close to the surface of the skin. This process leads to the self-limiting appearance of yellow papules. When diagnosing someone with eruptive xanthomas, it is important to measure their lipid and triglyceride levels. Patients with eruptive xanthomas may experience further

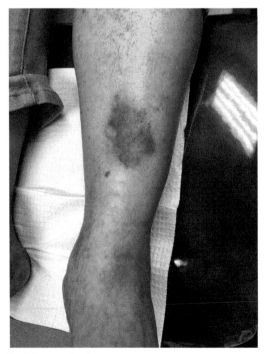

Fig. 1. Necrobiosis lipoidica on the leg.

complications like coronary artery disease and pancreatitis.[7] To avoid these complications, nutritional changes with the addition of fibrates or niacin to lower triglyceride levels should be prescribed (**Fig. 2**).

ACANTHOSIS NIGRICANS

Occurring in intertriginous areas as lesions of hyperchromic skin thickening, acanthosis nigricans is one of the most common cutaneous manifestations of chronic type 2 DM.[8] The most common area affected in children is the back of the neck.[9] Acanthosis nigricans is caused by hyperinsulinemia, leading to type 1 insulin growth factor synthesis by keratinocytes and fibroblasts, resulting in epidermal acanthosis nigricans. In obese patients, acanthosis nigricans coincides with metabolic syndrome. The main treatment is weight loss and physical exercise, although topical emollients with a urea base have been shown to be beneficial as well.[10]

Sixty-two percent of children presenting with acanthosis nigricans also had high insulin resistance; therefore, acanthosis nigricans can be used as a screening method to identify children at risk for type 2 DM.[9] Facial acanthosis nigricans, a subtype, occurs as a velvety thickening of skin most commonly on the forehead. The facial subtype presents more commonly in males with a positive oral glucose tolerance test, and an increased body mass index and waist to hip ratio.[11] It is noteworthy that smoking serves as a protective factor in the development of the facial subtype of acanthosis nigricans.[11]

DIABETIC DERMOPATHY

Diabetic dermopathy is known as the most common cutaneous manifestation of DM.[12,13] Diabetic dermopathy presents as well-defined hyperpigmented atrophic

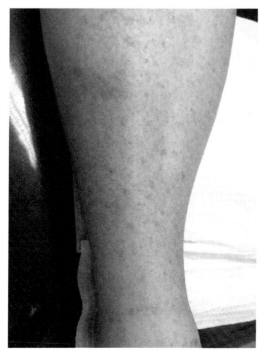

Fig. 2. Eruptive xanthoma on the legs.

depressions or papules, usually on the anterior tibia. Diabetic dermopathy results from the deposition of hemosiderin and/or melanin in the dermis.[12] Increased capillary basement membrane thickening has also been noted. It has been linked to be associated with neuropathy, nephropathy, and retinopathy.[13] (**Fig. 3**)

PERIUNGUAL TELANGIECTASIA

Periungual telangiectasia occurs owing to the loss of capillary loops as well as the dilation of the remaining capillaries. Periungual telangiectasia presents in nearly one-half of all patients with type 1 DM. It presents clinically as erythematous nail folds, fingertip or toe tenderness, and uneven cuticles.[14]

VITILIGO VULGARIS

Vitiligo vulgaris is more commonly seen in patients with type 1 diabetes. It appears clinically as hypopigmented skin patches. The mechanism between the association of vitiligo vulgaris and DM is unclear; however, it is theorized that polyglandular autoimmune syndrome plays a role.[14] Unfortunately, there is no definitive treatment for vitiligo vulgaris and current treatments have been proven unsatisfactory. Patients are advised to avoid direct sunlight and use sunscreen. In addition, topical corticosteroids can be used for localized vitiligo vulgaris. For more widespread generalized vitiligo vulgaris, UVB light treatment can be helpful.[14]

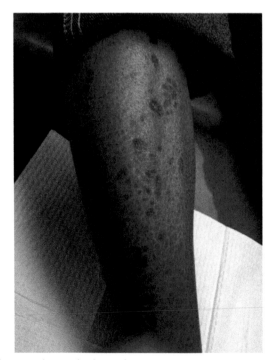

Fig. 3. diabetic dermopathy on the lower leg.

LICHEN PLANUS

Lichen planus presents as polygonal erythematous flat lesions and is frequently seen in both type 1 and type 2 diabetic patients. The lesions often appear on the wrist, the dorsum of the feet, and the lower legs. Oral lichen planus is also commonly seen and appears as white stripes known as Wickham's striae with a reticular pattern. Lichen planus affects both men and women equally. The treatment for lichen planus consists of topical corticosteroids or cyclosporine.[14]

PSORIASIS

Psoriasis is a common skin condition with the hallmark presentation of a red plaque with a silvery scale. Psoriasis can be a part of the metabolic syndrome. The metabolic syndrome is associated with a variety of maladies of the body owing to its indiscriminate inflammation of organ systems. One of its pertinent associations is with DM. There have been different reports on whether psoriasis can be used as an indicator of DM. One study revealed that 16% of patients with psoriasis had DM versus 6% in the control group, which was deemed clinically insignificant.[13] In this same study, 30% of the psoriatic group had DM, whereas 8% had it in the control group, which was deemed a significant finding. The key lessons that have been learned for various studies is that psoriasis has been correlated with the metabolic syndrome, and patients with psoriasis have often altered their lifestyles to decrease activity. Physicians need to be aware that patients with psoriasis may be at risk for DM, and so it is important to emphasize that diet and exercise must be continued at healthy levels to avoid the development of type 2 DM[13] (**Fig. 4**).

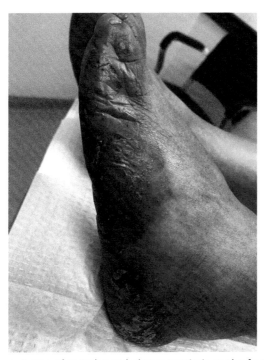

Fig. 4. A mixed presentation of pustular and plaque psoriasis on the foot of a patient with diabetes.

DIABETES AND NAILS

In patients with DM, the nails can be affected by a myriad of pathologies, including but not limited to fungal infections, yeast infections, neuropathy, and circulation issues. Nail pathologies can have a negative health impact in patients with DM. Although a cracked nail may seem insignificant, it can have disastrous effects in a patient with uncontrolled or advanced DM. Nail pathologies should be addressed and treated as soon as possible before they lead to complications. Nail proteins in patients with DM are associated with high rates of glycosylation.[15] This glycosylation weakens the immune system and allows for nail infections and nail breakdown to occur in patients with poorly controlled DM.[15,16]

Fungal infection of nails, also called onychomycosis, can be caused by the 3 groups of dermatophytes, *Microsporum*, *Epidermophyton*, and *Trichophyton*.[16] The most common infecting organism from the 3 classes is *Trichophyton rubrum*, which most commonly affects toenails, specifically the first and fifth toenails.[16] Fingernails can be infected as well, but the offending organisms for fingernails are usually *Tinea corporis* or *Tinea capitis*.[16] Onychomycosis presents as yellow or brown discoloration with thin, easily crumbled nails.[15] This distinct appearance of nails is important to a clinician because it can be used as a predictor for diabetic foot ulcer.[15] The treatment of onychomycosis is important because, without treatment, the infection in a diseased nail can spread to the surrounding skin, which can predispose the patient to ulcers, gangrene, and osteomyelitis.[16] The treatment of onychomycosis involves many options, with topical or oral medications available. Some topical medications to consider are efinaconazole, tavaborole, or ciclopirox.[16] Oral antifungal agents include terbinafine, itraconazole, or ultra-microsized griseofulvin.[16] The best treatment option should be determined by the clinician based on several factors, such as patient age, sex, weight, and overall wellness.[16]

In addition to the issues caused by glycosylation, the nervous and vascular systems can have an impact on nail growth. Neuropathy, a common DM complication, also may affect the nails. Because nail growth is constant, neuropathy can impair it, which can eventually lead to gait disturbances and neuropathic ulcers.[15] Neuropathic nails can present with yellow discoloration and a brittle texture.[15] Vascular issues can also impact nails. Vascular issues are common in people with DM owing to the glycation of capillaries.[17] Nails need a constant vascular supply, but vascular disease decreases circulation to the nail, which may lead to onycholysis.[15] Nails can also become distorted or thickened, which causes gait disturbances and can further lead to plantar neuropathic ulcers. A complete absence of circulation leads to nail matrix death, causing the whole nail to lyse and be shed.[15]

GRANULOMA ANNULARE

Granuloma annulare is a rare noninfectious inflammatory disorder of idiopathic origin. This condition is defined by mucin deposition, collagen degeneration, and interstitial histiocytes.[18,19] Although several clinical variants of this disease exist, only the generalized form shows a significant correlation to DM. The generalized granuloma annulare variant presents as several, small, firm, erythematous or skin-colored dermal papules distributed symmetrically on distal extremities and sun-exposed areas of the trunk. These individual lesions gradually expand and involute centrally, coalescing into annular plaques with indurated borders. Although generalized granuloma annulare is only prevalent in about 0.3% of diabetics, studies show that 21% to 77% of patients with generalized granuloma annulare have type 2 DM. Progression of this disorder tends to be persistent and relapsing especially in individuals with high glucose levels[10] (**Fig. 5**).

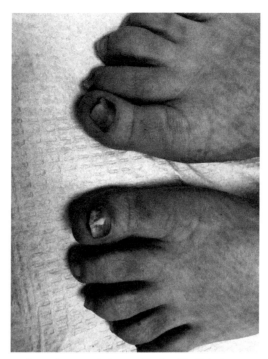

Fig. 5. Distal subungual onychomycosis in a patient with diabetes.

SCLEREDEMA DIABETICORUM

Scleredema diabeticorum is a rare chronic connective tissue condition characterized by asymptomatic thickening of the dermis, which is usually localized to the upper back, shoulders, and posterior neck with acral sparing. The thickened skin is indurated and erythematous and may have a peau d'orange appearance. Severe cases may present with pain and decreased mobility.[10,18] Scleredema diabeticorum is noted in 2.5% to 14.0% of patients with type 2 DM, with the highest prevalence in obese adult males exhibiting poor glycemic control and long-standing DM.[20] The pathogenesis of scleredema diabeticorum is believed to be associated with nonenzymatic glycosylation of collagen which may interfere with collagen degradation, resulting in subsequent accumulation.[18,20]

SUMMARY

Owing to the systemic and local effects of DM, a wide array of skin conditions may be seen throughout the body, but also specifically on the lower extremity. It is pertinent for the practitioner to be aware of these conditions to counsel the patient, prevent complications, and create a treatment plan.

CLINICS CARE POINTS

- Nail issues in patients with diabetes should be addressed, diagnosed, and managed.
- Patients with psoriasis and diabetes should be monitored for the metabolic syndrome as they are at higher risk for cardiovascular events.

• Bullosis diabeticorum are blisters that may form on the lower extremity often without inflammation. These may recur over time.

REFERENCES

1. Huntley AC. The cutaneous manifestations of diabetes mellitus. J Am Acad Dermatol 1989;&:427–55.
2. Tecilazick F, Kafanas A, Veves A. Cutaneous alterations in diabetes mellitus. Wounds 2011;23(7):192–203.
3. Karadag A, Ozlu E, Lavery M. Cutaneous manifestations of diabetes mellitus and the metabolic syndrome. Clin Dermatol 2018;36:89–93.
4. Duff M, Demidova O, Blackburn S, et al. Cutaneous manifestations of diabetes mellitus. Clin Diabetes 2015;33(1):40–8.
5. Rosen J, Yosipovitch G. Skin manifestations of diabetes mellitus. In: Endotext [Internet]. South Dartmouth, MA: MDText.com, Inc; 2000.
6. Goodheart H, Burk P. Cutaneous manifestations of systemic disease. Plastic Surgery Key; 2016. Available at: https://plasticsurgerykey.com/cutaneous-manifestations-of-systemic-disease/.
7. Morgan AJ1, Schwartz RA. Diabetic dermopathy: a subtle sign with grave implications. J Am Acad Dermatol 2008;58(3):447–51.
8. Mendes AL, Miot HA, Haddad VJ. Diabetes mellitus and the skin. An Bras Dermatol 2017;92(1):8–20.
9. Bhagyanathan M, Dhayanithy D, Parambath VA, et al. Acanthosis nigricans: a screening test for insulin resistance – an important risk factor for diabetes mellitus type-2. J Fam Med Prim Care 2017;6(1):43–6.
10. Murphy-Chutorian B, Han G, Cohen SR. Dermatologic manifestations of diabetes mellitus. Endocrinol Metab Clin North Am 2013;42(4):869–98.
11. Panda S, Das A, Lahiri K, et al. Facial acanthosis nigricans: a morphological marker of metabolic syndrome. Indian J Dermatol 2017;62(6):591–7.
12. McCash S, Emanuel PO. Defining diabetic dermopathy. J Dermatol 2011;38:988–92.
13. Khunger N, Gupta D, Ramesh V. Is psoriasis a new cutaneous marker for metabolic syndrome? A study in Indian patients. Indian J Dermatol 2013;58(4):313–4.
14. Simone H, AArt B, Thio H. Skin manifestations of diabetes. Cleve Clin J Med 2008;75(11):772–86.
15. Hillson R. Nails in diabetes. Pract Diabetes 2017;34(7):230–1.
16. Eisman S, Sinclair R. Fungal nail infection: diagnosis and management. Br Med J 2014;348(7951):27.
17. Makrantonaki E, Jiang D, Hossini A, et al. Diabetes mellitus and the skin. Rev Endocr Metab Disord 2016;17(3):269–82.
18. Horton W, Boler P, Subauste A. Diabetes mellitus and the skin: recognition and management of cutaneous manifestations. South Med J 2016;109(10):636–46.
19. Nambiar K, Jagadeesan S, Balasubramanian P, et al. Successful treatment of generalized granuloma annulare with pentoxifylline. Indian Dermatol Online J 2017;8(3):218.
20. Levy L, Zeichner J. Dermatologic manifestation of diabetes. J Diabetes 2012;4(1):68–76.

Pyoderma Gangrenosum

A Literature Review

Madeleine Barbe, DPM, Andrea Batra, DPM,
Stephanie Golding, DPM, Olivia Hammond, DPM,
Jacqueline C. Higgins, DPM, Amber O'Connor, DPM,
Tracey C. Vlahovic, DPM*

KEYWORDS

- Pyoderma gangrenosum • Neutrophilic dermatoses • Leg ulcer

KEY POINTS

- PG is a neutrophilic dermatosis that often occurs on the lower extremity.
- It is characteristically painful and may present with other disease states.
- If it occurs with an associated disease, it is important to treat the underlying disease state.

INTRODUCTION

Pyoderma gangrenosum (PG) is a rare inflammatory skin disease that is classified as a neutrophilic dermatosis.[1–4] It has a classic presentation of rapidly progressive, severely painful ulcers,[1,3–7] which are frequently found in the lower extremity.[3–5,7,8] PG is often seen in patients with other systemic illnesses, most commonly inflammatory bowel disease (IBD).[2,3,6,8] Associated diseases often share the element of neutrophil dysfunction.[2,9]

Although many aspects of PG's pathogenesis remain unclear,[1,2,4,5,7,8,10] it is thought to be multifactorial.[2,4,5] Although it can be idiopathic, abnormalities in the immune system and in the inflammatory response may contribute.[1,2,4,6] Genetic predisposition can also play a role,[1,4,11] and there have been rare familial syndromes involving PG.[2,4–6]

There is often a delay in diagnosis because there are no specific laboratory markers or assessments that can confirm PG.[4–7] It is a diagnosis of exclusion,[1,4–7] and suspected individuals should get skin biopsies and other work-ups to rule out underlying or coexisting conditions. Although there are no officially approved criteria for diagnosis, there have been suggested guidelines that require a rapidly progressing ulcer with violaceous and undermined borders, as well as ruling out other causes of

Conflict of interest: None of the authors have any financial interests to disclose for this article.
Temple University School of Podiatric Medicine, 148 North 8th Street, Philadelphia, PA 19107, USA
* Corresponding author.
E-mail address: traceyv@temple.edu

cutaneous ulceration. The suggested guidelines also propose that 2 minor conditions should be met, which may include history of pathergy or cribriform scarring, systemic disease associated with PG, certain histopathology findings, or a rapid treatment response to systemic steroids.[4–6] Histopathology should show neutrophilic infiltrate[1,4,5,10] without signs of infection or significant vasculopathy.[4]

Other than the most common classic ulcerative form of PG, there are several variants: pustular, bullous, vegetative, and superficial granulomatous (**Fig. 1**). The classic ulcerative form starts as sterile pustules that quickly progresses into an erythematous, violaceous, necrotic ulcer. Bullous PG, common on the face and upper extremities, has quickly evolving vesicles that coalesce into large bullae, without necrosis or cribriform scarring. Pustular PG has sterile pustules that may resolve or ulcerate; this variant is highly associated with IBD. The vegetative form is the most uncommon and benign.[4–6]

There is still much to be discovered about appropriate treatments for the disease, and currently there is no gold standard. However, depending on the severity of PG, certain medications are routinely used. If the lesions are rapidly evolving, it is recommended to use systemic steroids at moderate to high doses.[4,5] When PG is indolent, topical or intralesional therapy may be sufficient.[2,6] It is also important to provide wound care to keep the area clean.[1,4] Certain researchers have suggested gentle, cautious debridement,[1,6] but this cannot be confidently advocated because it is a controversial method. Because of the pathergy phenomenon that is seen in many PG cases, debridement can increase the risk of further damage and worsen the ulceration[2,4] (**Fig. 2**).

PG has a poor prognosis[4,8,11] and can be devastating because of the pain inflicted and the diminished quality of life of those affected.[11] Further scientific understanding

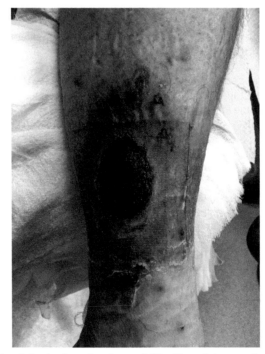

Fig. 1. An example of classic ulcerative form of PG with a violaceous border.

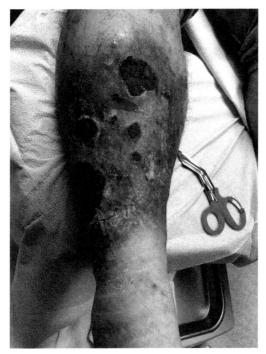

Fig. 2. An example of pathergy following aggressive debridement of the original wound.

of the disease process will increase physician understanding of PG, allowing quicker diagnosis and increasingly targeted therapy.[2]

HISTORY

PG was first described in 1908 by Louis Brocq, a French dermatologist who called the lesions geometric phagedenism. Geometric referred to the pattern commonly seen on PG ulcer edges, and phagedenism described the rapidly progressive nature.[4] In 1930, Brunsting and colleagues began using the term PG.[1,5] They originally believed it was caused by infectious dissemination from a distant site.[5] However, it is now known that PG is unrelated to infection,[1,4,7,11] although superinfection can occur at the site of the lesion.[4,11] The first large series of patients that presented with PG occurred in 1957. Nineteen patients had similar PG lesions and it was considered a dermatologic emergency.[5] Because cortisone was discovered in 1950, it has been somewhat effective in managing PG, but rebound often occurs,[5] because it is a chronic, recalcitrant disease.[1,4] Physicians now prescribe higher doses of cortisone in an attempt to prevent recurrence.[9] The suggested guidelines for diagnosis, although not confirmed definitively, were first developed in 2004.[4] These guidelines support commonalities seen in many patients with PG.

EPIDEMIOLOGY

It is estimated that PG affects 3 to 10 individuals per million each year worldwide,[6,8] but this may be undercounted because of the difficulty in diagnosing.[1,7,12] A retrospective cohort study done in 2012 found that the median age at presentation was

59 years,[8] although many studies support a broad range of age of onset.[1,4] The same study[8] found that there is an increased incidence of PG ulcerations in both children and the elderly, whereas a more recent study[4] done in 2015 has shown PG to have an onset in middle-aged adults and only a 4% incidence in children. In a 2018 study by Ashchyan and colleagues,[3] a random patient set was gathered between the years 2000 and 2016, and most participants were white (84.8%) and female (75%). There have been numerous studies supporting that overweight white women are at a greater risk of developing the disease than their counterparts.[3,4,8]

CAUSE AND PATHOGENESIS

PG has a multifactorial cause and pathogenesis.[1,4,5] The current body of research supports 3 main mechanisms contributing to cause PG: abnormal production of inflammatory cytokines, neutrophil dysfunction, and specific gene mutations.[2] Understanding the disease process of PG will help in early recognition of at-risk patients and will help physicians and researchers develop targeted and personalized treatments.[2]

Inflammation

Inflammatory dysregulation and autoinflammation are thought to play a key role in the onset of PG.[2] Proliferation and infiltration of clonal T cells at the PG ulcer edges and cytokine abundance within lesions lead to active recruitment of neutrophils.[4,6]

T cells are implicated in the development of PG because of the discovery of oligoclonal T-cell expansion both in the serum and in the ulcer edges in patients with PG. Cluster of differentiation (CD) 3+ T cells and CD163+ macrophages were the primary cells found in the wound edges of 21 PG ulcers studied.[2] Increased numbers of T-helper (Th) 17 cells and low numbers of regulatory T cells has also been observed in PG ulcers.[4] Interleukin (IL)-17 antagonists have been proposed as a treatment of PG in patients found to have this imbalance of T-regulatory cells and Th17 cells.[2] Medications that affect T-cell function or induce T-cell apoptosis, such as alefacept and visilizumab, have been effective in treating PG ulcers, further supporting the role of T cells in PG.[2]

Abnormal cytokine signaling by these infiltrating T cells and macrophages is likely a component of the disease process.[6] Commonly reported inflammatory mediators found to be at increased levels in PG lesions are IL-8, IL-17, IL-23, and tumor necrosis factor alpha (TNF-α).[2,9] High levels of IL-8, a potent chemotactic factor for neutrophils, are found in the PG wound bed.[2,5] Th17 cells, which proliferate around the lesions, produce IL-17.[4] IL-23, a member of the IL-12 proinflammatory cytokine family, was found to be overexpressed in recalcitrant PG lesions.[2] IL-23 is an important component for activating neutrophils and stimulating other inflammatory factors.[6] IL-23 also boosts the expansion of Th17 cells. The human monoclonal antibody ustekinumab was effective in targeting IL-12 and IL-23 in several PG cases.[2]

In addition, a study comparing PG ulcers with healthy skin found overexpression of TNF-α; chemokines 1, 2, 3, and 16; matrix metalloproteinase (MMP) 2 and 9; and IL-1β. Increased levels of IL-1β and its receptor suggest that autoinflammation is occurring because of inflammasome creation. The inflammasome is a protein complex that is activated in an environment of stress or infection and promotes proliferation of inflammatory cytokines. Dysfunctional activation of the inflammasome in the absence of infection can initiate an inflammatory chain reaction leading to development of PG.[2]

Defects in the Janus kinase (JAK)– signal transducer and activator of transcription (STAT) pathway result in neutrophil proliferation and inflammation.[2,11] Granulocyte colony–stimulating factor (G-CSF) is an activator of the JAK-STAT pathway and plays a role in neutrophilic dermatoses such as PG, where it mediates adhesion and proliferation of neutrophils in sites of inflammation. Constitutive JAK2 activation, stimulated by G-CSF, provides growth and survival of hematopoietic clones, leading to myeloproliferative disorders and immune system modification.[13] G-CSF therapy has been reported to induce PG.[2,4]

In PG during pregnancy, several factors may provide a favorable inflammatory setting for PG development. Some cases have been explained by pathergy because the PG ulcer was at the site of cesarean section. In other cases, there was a patient history of systemic inflammatory disease. During pregnancy, there is a physiologic shift from balanced Th1 and Th2 activity to upregulated Th2 activity. Although Th2 can be protective against spontaneous abortion, preterm delivery, and preeclampsia, it produces many cytokines, of which GM-CSF is an attractant of neutrophilic inflammation.[2]

Immune dysfunction is shown by the presence of other immune-mediated comorbidities and a typical positive response to immunomodulatory drugs such as corticosteroids, anti–TNF-α modalities, and calcineurin inhibitors.[1,4,6] As the specific inflammatory mediators involved are elucidated, personalized therapy may be created.[2]

Neutrophil Dysfunction

PG is a neutrophilic dermatosis, a type of disorder characterized by skin lesions with heavy neutrophilic infiltrates without presence of infection.[2] Recent studies have shown that infiltration of neutrophils is caused by signaling from inflammatory mediators. The mechanisms of neutrophil dysfunction that have been observed include abnormal neutrophil chemotaxis, migration, phagocytosis, hyperactivity, and bactericidal ability.[2,4,5]

PG is associated with several diseases that also have a neutrophilic pathogenesis, further supporting the role of neutrophil dysfunction in PG pathogenesis. Some of these diseases include IBD, which has neutrophil infiltrates in intestinal tissue and stool, and rheumatoid arthritis and hematologic disorders, such as paraproteinemias, malignancies, and immunoglobulin A gammopathies, which have defects in chemotaxis.[2]

Approximately 20% to 30% of patients with PG show pathergy, a phenomenon where trauma such as debridement causes further ulceration and breakdown of the skin. Another disease where pathergy is a common source of ulceration, known as Behçet disease, has abundant neutrophils in its pathergic lesions, highlighting the significance of neutrophil dysfunction in pathergy, and therefore PG.[2]

Note that leukocyte adhesion deficiency type 1, an autosomal recessive disorder where defective adhesion to the vessel wall causes inability of neutrophils to extravasate from circulation into the tissue, has been discovered in patients with PG. With very few neutrophils able to reach the wound location in the tissue, these cases show that there are many other factors that contribute to development of PG and neutrophils are not acting alone.[2] This finding highlights the complexity of PG pathogenesis.

Genetics

There are several known genetic syndromes linked to PG. PAPA syndrome results from an autosomal dominant mutation of the PSTPIP-1 gene encoding CD-2–binding protein 1 on chromosome 15q. PAPA syndrome is characterized by a triad of pyogenic sterile arthritis, cystic acne, and PG.[2,5,11] A different mutation in the same PSTPIP-1 gene results in PAPASH syndrome, characterized by a tetrad of pyogenic sterile arthritis, PG, acne, and hidradenitis suppurativa. Similarly, PASH syndrome is characterized by PG, acne, and hidradenitis suppurativa, but does not have pyogenic arthritis. PASH syndrome is caused by an increase in microsatellite repeats of CCTG in the promoter of PSTPIP-1 and results in increased macrophage chemotaxis, extracellular matrix destruction, subsequent signaling for neutrophil infiltration, and worsening of PG lesions.[2,11] Excessive IL-1 and TNF-α production are thought to precipitate PAPA syndrome and its variants.[2,4,11] Normally, the PSTPIP-1–encoded protein binds to pyrin, which regulates inflammasomes. When this gene is mutated, there is excessive production of IL-1β by inflammasomes. Because of the pathophysiology, anakinra IL-1 receptor antagonist, TNF-α inhibitors, and canakinumab (a human monoclonal antibody to IL-1β) have been successful in treating PG in these syndromes.[11]

Specific gene loci are found in both PG and IBD, including IL-8RA, PR domain–containing protein 1 (PRDM1), and tissue inhibitor of metalloproteinase 3 (TIMP3).[2,11] The genetic loci of TRAF-interacting protein 2, which is associated with IBD, is also found to increase susceptibility to developing PG, erythema nodosum, and psoriasis.[2] JAK2 mutation in cases of PG leads to defective JAK-STAT pathway, as discussed earlier, causing inflammation.[11] The JAK1 and JAK2 inhibitor, ruxolitinib, healed chronic PG ulcers that were accompanied by polycythemia vera.[2,6] In addition, genetic predisposition is highlighted by a report of 6 families with a total of 14 members having PG but lacking any genetic abnormalities or criteria for a genetic syndrome.[2,11]

The current knowledge of the pathogenesis of PG can be summarized as a contribution of inflammatory mediator action, neutrophil dysfunction, and genetic predisposition, although PG is still considered to be poorly understood.[1,4,5,8] Continued investigation into the mechanisms of autoinflammation and specific mutations and inheritance patterns is needed to further elucidate the pathogenesis of PG and will help clinicians to develop effective therapies.[2,11]

DIAGNOSIS

Current research aims to turn PG from a diagnosis of exclusion[1,5,9,13] to a diagnosis with set inclusion criteria to confidently rule out a wide array of disorders. Differential diagnoses of PG are numerous and include infections of bacterial, mycobacterial, fungal, parasitic, and viral origins. Sweet syndrome, insect bites, cutaneous tumors, skin lymphomas, halogenoderma, and Behçet disease can all appear similar to PG.[4,14] Researchers have attempted to determine comorbidities, demographics, and presenting symptoms that are seen with PG more frequently than with other diagnoses. In the 2012 study conducted by Ashchyan and colleagues,[3] researchers compiled diagnostic data from the University of Pennsylvania health system, Brigham and Women's, and the Massachusetts General Hospitals from 2000 to 2015, in which they found records of 356 patients given a diagnosis of PG. Patient data were sorted into 2 groups: less than 65 years old and more than 65 years old. Researchers studied clinical presentations and comorbidities appearing in each group and found that there was a strong association of PG with IBD in patients less than 65 years old and that pathergy was found more often in patients more than 65 years old. The researchers also found strong positive correlations with rheumatoid arthritis, ankylosing spondylitis, solid organ malignant neoplasms, malignant hematologic neoplasms, and several other hematologic disorders.[3] Although there were strong associations with comorbidities found in this study, all of the patients' data were taken from tertiary centers in 2 cities, which may have an impact on demographics and the prevalence of certain comorbidities. This information does not lead to a specific set of diagnostic criteria, but it does suggest correlated diagnoses that can be evaluated to increase the index of suspicion that a patient may have PG.

A 2018 study conducted by Maverakis and colleagues[7] set out to determine a specific set of diagnostic criteria for PG. This study, done by researchers at the University of California, Davis, was conducted as a Delphi consensus exercise. Questionnaires were sent to 15 physicians from 6 countries and 10 universities, and 12 of the physicians participated in the exercise. Physicians were selected based on history of major publications in well-known medical journals. The responses to multiple rounds of questioning were tabulated and researchers determined major and minor criteria for the diagnosis of PG. Physicians in the study agreed that biopsy containing neutrophilic infiltrate was the major criterion that must be present for a diagnosis of PG. In addition, 4 minor criteria (of the 8 the panel discussed) must also be present to confirm the diagnosis. Minor criteria included findings such as histologic exclusion of infection, pathergy, history of IBD or arthritis, papule or pustule that rapidly ulcerates, multiple ulcerations with at least 1 occurring on the lower extremity, cribriform scars at healed sites, erythematous ulcers with undermining borders, and a decrease in ulcer size following immunosuppressive treatment.[7]

Further research performed by Su and colleagues[5] attempted to develop diagnostic criteria for bullous, pustular, and vegetative PG subtypes and supports the conclusion by Maverakis and colleagues[7] that specific major and minor criteria can lead physicians to a concise diagnosis. Determination of what are major versus minor criteria differs based on PG classification. For each subtype, researchers determined that diagnosis can be made after PG presents with 2 major and at least 2 minor criteria. According to Su and colleagues,[5] the major criteria for bullous PG include painful, inflammatory bullae that enlarge rapidly and coalesce, and exclusion of other causes of bullae. The minor criteria include histopathology showing neutrophilic infiltrate and subepidermal bullae with or without epidermal necrosis, associated hematologic malignancy, pathergy, and positive response to steroids. Like a diagnosis of bullous PG, the diagnosis of pustular PG requires that both major criteria and at least 2 of the minor criteria determined in the study be met for diagnosis. Major criteria for pustular PG include painful pustules with a surrounding halo and that other causes of pustules have been excluded. Minor criteria include neutrophilic infiltrate on histopathologic investigation, associated IBD, and improvement of PG with control of IBD. For a diagnosis of vegetative PG, researchers determined that major criteria included chronic erythematous plaques with sinus formation and shallow, uncomfortable ulcerations or erosions and an exclusion of other causes of vegetative lesions. Minor criteria for vegetative PG included dermal and histiocytic dermal infiltrate, no associated disease, and a positive response to minor treatment measures.[5]

Current research on the diagnosis of PG suggests that certain presentations and comorbidities should be used as diagnostic criteria despite the lack of specific laboratory tests[5] and laboratory markers for diagnosis.[9,14] A complete work-up should include extensive blood and urine screening, biopsy of border and adjacent skin, and a colonoscopy[9,13] to include or exclude the diagnosis of PG. Once a diagnosis of PG is suspected or confirmed, subtyping can be achieved following the categorization guidelines set forth by Su and colleagues[5] to determine prognosis and tailor treatment.

ASSOCIATED DISEASE STATES

Because of the difficult nature of diagnosing PG, it is important to discuss some of the comorbidities to help give clues during assessment. PG is often idiopathic but has been found to be associated with systemic diseases in more than 50% of cases.[8] In the most recent comorbidity study done by Ashchyan and colleagues,[3] the association with systemic disease has increased to 66.3%, the most common being IBD (41%) with an equal association of ulcerative colitis and Crohn disease. Additional associations include inflammatory arthritis, rheumatoid arthritis, psoriatic arthritis, and ankylosing spondylitis (20.5%), solid organ malignant neoplasms (6.5%), hematologic malignant neoplasms (5.9%), and hematologic disorders, including monoclonal gammopathy of undetermined significance, myelodysplastic syndrome, and polycythemia vera (4.8%).[3] Although having one of the associated diseases does not confirm a PG diagnosis, it can be useful knowing that there is a higher incidence of these diseases in patients with PG, compared with other illnesses. This knowledge may help guide physicians toward gathering the correct diagnostic data.

Following the evidence that PG is highly correlated with IBD, especially in patients less than 65 years of age, it is recommended to lower the threshold to involve a gastroenterology work-up in young patients that present with PG, including endoscopy and colonoscopy.[3] The 2 most common dermatologic manifestations of IBD are PG and erythema nodosum. It is suspected that the inappropriate immune activation that causes IBD also leads to the cutaneous ulcerations and redness seen in those 2 diseases.[10] Patients more than 65 years of age are also at risk of underlying IBD, but they are more likely to present with a hematologic disorder, and therefore a complete hematologic work-up is highly recommended.[3]

CLINICAL PRESENTATION

PG most frequently affects the lower extremities.[3,5] Seventy-eight percent of PG ulcers occur on the lower leg,[1] with the most common location being the pretibial area.[4] Other areas may also be involved, including the trunk, arms, peristomal sites, head and neck, and stomal sites, in that order from most to least common.[1,8] The perineum is rarely involved, but can be a more common site in children. PG has the potential to involve any cutaneous site on the body.[5]

Typically, PG has a rapid onset, although it can be variable.[4,8] The lesions begin as tender papules, papulopustules, or vesicles that then progress rapidly into painful, enlarging ulcers.[3,4] Without including the inflamed but intact skin surrounding them, the average size of PG lesions is 54 × 36 mm.[1] The clinical presentation and changes seen correlate with the age of the lesion.[5]

Severe pain, a common symptom, is out of proportion to the size of the ulcer.[1,3,5,6,8] Systemic symptoms may also occur and can include fever, joint pain, malaise, and myalgia.[4,6]

The classic ulcerative form of PG presents as a nodule or sterile pustule that progresses into a necrotic, mucopurulent ulcer.[5] The border of the ulcer is edematous, violaceous, undermined, serpiginous, and expanding, because of the dynamic process of liquefactive necrosis.[1,3,5] There are 2 distinct stages of the classic ulcerative form of PG that are described in the literature: the active ulcerative stage and the wound-healing stage. In the active ulcerative stage, the ulcer presents with an erythematous, inflammatory halo surrounding it and raised edges with an undermining border.[4] The halo is typically 1 to 2 cm surrounding the lesion and represents involved skin that is not yet necrotic.[5] At this stage, the ulcer itself can be necrotic. In the wound-healing stage, the Gulliver sign is present. The Gulliver sign is described as stringlike projections of epithelium around the edges of the ulcer that straddle the border between the ulcer bed and the normal skin around the lesion. These lesions are aseptic, but there is a chance of superinfection.[4] Older and subsiding lesions may heal with a thin cribriform scar.[5] This feature is of minor importance in the diagnosis of PG, because it simply supports the diagnosis, but can be of major importance in the patient's quality of life, because the scar can lead to disfigurement.[4,5] A poor prognosis is associated with the classic ulcerative form of PG.[4]

Bullous PG is one of the variant forms of the disease.[4–6] It is found on the upper extremities, such as the dorsal surfaces of the hands and extensor regions of the arms, and on the face and head.[4,8] The bullous form presents with rapidly evolving, painful vesicles and enlarging bullae that can group and coalesce. The bullae have a shallow erosion in the center that is necrotic, but they are not necrotic ulcers like the classic ulcerative form. The surrounding tissue can have an erythematous halo or be gray.[4,5] On histologic examination, dermal neutrophilia and subepidermal bullae are present. In 70% of cases of this variant form of PG, the disease is associated with a hematologic malignancy.[5] When this association is present, this can be a sign of malignant transformation and often results in a poor prognosis and more aggressive disease for the patient.[4] It is common to see this variant in patients with lymphoproliferative diseases as a paraneoplastic phenomenon, and there can be overlap with the neutrophilic disorder known as Sweet syndrome.[4,6] Uniquely, there is no cribriform scarring with the bullous form of PG.[5]

Pustular PG is another variant form of the disease. This form presents as many pustules that either resolve or become ulcerated.[6] The pustules are sterile and are surrounded with an erythematous halo.[3,4] Typically, this variant appears on the trunk or extensor surfaces of the limbs.[4] Pustular PG is associated with IBD and may be a marker of activity of the bowel disease of the patient.[4–6] This form of PG often improves when the underlying IBD is treated.[4,5]

Vegetative or superficial granulomatous PG is the final variant form of the disease. This type is the most rare and benign, because it is localized, limited, and responds well to less aggressive forms of treatment. Vegetative PG is less often associated with systemic disorders than the other variants are. The lesions are verrucous and ulcerative but do not have an undermined border. Progression of this form is slow and contrasts with the rapid progression of the classic ulcerative form.[4,5] On histologic examination, granuloma formation and sinus tracts are present.[5] The granulomas have 3 layers: a center with neutrophilic inflammation, surrounding palisading histiocytes, and a rim of lymphocytic infiltrate. More than 1 of these subtypes of PG may be present in the same patient.[4]

The phenomenon of pathergy is seen in approximately 30% of patients with PG.[1,3–6] A pathergy skin test can be performed, which involves poking the skin of the patient and observing for an exaggerated response to the injury.[6] PG ulcers that present with pathergy are often made worse by surgery, and a common recommendation is to avoid surgical debridement of these lesions.[4]

A chronic, relapsing course can occur in patients with PG.[4] In a retrospective review published in 2011, 65% of patients with PG had 2 or more ulcers at some point in the 8 years over which the study was conducted. Thirty percent of patients with PG have 3 or more ulcers during the same flare of the disease, as reported in the same study.[1]

In a study that compared PG with chronic venous ulceration, pathergy, purulent discharge, and craterlike holes that showed cribriform scarring later on were unique to patients with PG. These presentations were not seen in any patients with chronic venous ulcerations. Approximately half of the patients with PG in this study presented with pustules, but no patients with chronic venous ulceration had this presentation.[14] It is important to note these differences in clinical presentation when trying to diagnose a patient that has these differential diagnoses.

PROGNOSIS

According to a retrospective cohort study published in 2012, the risk of death for patients with PG is 3 times higher than for the general population and almost 2 times higher than for patients with IBD without PG. Despite patients' often numerous comorbidities, adjusting for these did not eliminate the increased mortalities associated with PG.[8] With the associated risk of death this high, the importance of properly identifying and treating this disease should not be underestimated.

Previous case reports and case series have reported mortalities of 30%,[8] whereas another retrospective study of 103 patients found that, in an 8-year period, the mortality associated with PG was 16%. This same retrospective review, published in 2011, found that the mean age of death in the patients with PG was 67 years, and the main causes of death were heart failure, renal failure, and hematological comorbidities.[1]

Bullous PG, one of a few subtypes of the disease, can be particularly lethal in patients with leukemia or polycythemia rubra vera.[5] Finding bullous PG in these patients is an ominous sign, because they tend to develop progressive and unresponsive hematologic malignancies and die within a short period of the appearance of the disease.[1]

For patients with PG who survive, the disease has a significant effect on their quality of life. PG can lead to scarring, pain, functional impairment, and bacterial superinfection.[11] These potential outcomes of the disease can create extensive challenges for patients and notably diminish their overall quality of life.

TREATMENT

Because PG is a disease with many contributing factors, it is important to treat the underlying disease and tailor therapy to the patient's specific condition.[6] Therefore, there is no gold standard way of treating PG. Treatment usually involves a combination of wound management, dressings, and both topical and systemic agents.[1]

It is important to clean wounds to prevent infection. Debridement must be done carefully, although it is not commonly recommended because of the pathergy phenomenon, followed up by local wound management.[1] Grafting and compression should only be done on ulcers that are not infected or inflamed, and should be done in conjunction with immunosuppressants.[4] Dressing the wounds is also important because most wounds have exudate.[5]

For patients with milder disease, topical and intralesional steroids or topical tacrolimus alone have been shown to be effective,[4,6] as have topical dapsone and sulfapyridine.[5] However, most patients require more than solely topical agents. The most prescribed agent is an oral corticosteroid such as prednisone, followed by topical steroids.[3]

Systemic corticosteroids, such as prednisone, have been shown to be effective in rapidly growing lesions. Remarkably, pain subsides in 48 to 72 hours in those patients.[5] In addition, 96% of patients were found to respond to steroid treatment.[9] Although widely used, 1 study found that prednisone performed the worst of all agents unless started early and at high doses.[9] Other studies, such as the STOP GAP study, compared prednisolone and cyclosporine and found them to be equally efficacious.[6] Although both are commonly used, the severe side effects of prednisolone, such as infection and bowel perforation, and of cyclosporine, such as kidney injury and ruptured abdominal aortic aneurysm, have led doctors to branch out and explore other agents to add as a combination therapy to the classically used ones.[9]

Biologic agents have been incorporated into PG ulcer treatment in recent years and have had success across the board. Infliximab, a TNF-α inhibitor, was shown to be so

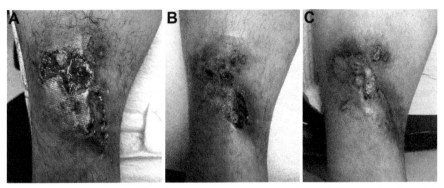

Fig. 3. (*A*) First visit; (*B*) starting the systemic therapy apremilast; (*C*) 1 year after first visit.

effective that the clinical trial ended early, and all patients were switched to infliximab. Eighty-nine percent of participants benefited in 6 weeks. The same study found that 100% of patients with PG and IBD improved with infliximab.[9] Because T cells are thought to play a role in the pathogenesis of PG, biologics such as alefacept and visilizumab have also been useful in some cases.[2] Other biologics, such as ruxolitinib,[13] adalimumab,[9] anakinra,[2] ustekinumab, canakinumab, tocilizumab,[6] and etanercept,[1] have also been shown to heal PG ulcers, depending on patient comorbidities (**Fig. 3**).

Other treatments that have worked in some patients include oral dapsone,[3] B vitamins,[11] and other immunosuppressive agents such as thalidomide[14] and azathioprine.[9] Antimicrobials have had mixed success, likely because of the presence or absence of infection, with some studies showing that they were effective in diminishing ulcer size[5] and others showing no significant effect.[4]

When treatment is working, patients have decreased pain and erythema, diminishing ulcer sizes,[5] and decreased white and red blood cell counts.[13] The literature agrees that a combination of approaches works best in healing patients with PG, and therapy can be tailored to patients based specifically on the makeup of their disease.

SUMMARY

Overall, this literature review focused on compiling the history, cause, diagnosis, presentation, prognosis, and treatment of PG. Although PG has been a focus of recent research, it is still not completely understood. Many comorbidities of this multifactorial disease have been identified, but it is still unclear why some patients get the disease and others do not. Future studies should focus on predictive factors, because identifying predictors before ulceration occurs could influence rates of healing, relapse, and prognosis for patients.

REFERENCES

1. Binus AM, Qureshi AA, Li VW, et al. Pyoderma gangrenosum: a retrospective review of patient Characteristics, comorbidities and therapy in 103 patients. Br J Dermatol 2011;165(6):1244–50. Available at: https://www.ncbi.nlm.nih.gov/pubmed/21824126. Accessed April 1, 2018.

2. Braswell SF, Kostopoulos TC, Ortega-Loayza AG, et al. Pathophysiology of pyoderma gangrenosum (PG): and updated review. J Am Acad Dermatol 2015;73(4):

691–8. Available at: https://www-sciencedirect-com.libproxy.temple.edu/science/article/pii/S0190962215017661#bib17. Accessed March 10, 2018.

3. Ashchyan HJ, Butler DC, Nelson CA, et al. The association of age with clinical presentation and comorbidities of pyoderma gangrenosum. JAMA Dermatol 2018. https://doi.org/10.1001/jamadermatol.2017.5978. Available at: https://www.ncbi.nlm.nih.gov/pubmed/29450453. Accessed March 10, 2018.

4. Gameiro A, Pereira N, Cardoso JC, et al. Pyoderma gangrenosum: challenges and solutions. Clin Cosmet Investig Dermatol 2015;8:285–93. Available at: https://www.ncbi.nlm.nih.gov/pmc/articles/PMC4454198/. Accessed March 10, 2018.

5. Su WPD, Davis MDP, Weenig RH, et al. Pyoderma gangrenosum: clinicopathologic correlation and proposed diagnostic criteria. Int J Dermatol 2004;43(11): 790–800. Available at: https://www.ncbi.nlm.nih.gov/pubmed/15533059. Accessed April 1, 2018.

6. Schmieder SJ, Krishnamurthy K. Pyoderma gangrenosum. In: StatPearls. Treasure Island (FL): StatPearls Publishing; 2018. Available at: https://www.ncbi.nlm.nih.gov/books/NBK482223/. Accessed March 10, 2018.

7. Maverakis E, Ma C, Shinkai K, et al. Diagnostic criteria of ulcerative pyoderma gangrenosum. JAMA Dermatol 2018. https://doi.org/10.1001/jamadermatol.2017.5980. Available at: https://jamanetwork-com.libproxy.temple.edu/journals/jamadermatology/fullarticle/2672271. Accessed March 10, 2018.

8. Langan SM, Groves RW, Card TR, et al. Incidence, mortality, and disease associations of pyoderma gangrenosum in the United Kingdom: a Retrospective Cohort Study. J Invest Dermatol 2012;132(9):2166–70. Available at: https://www.ncbi.nlm.nih.gov/pubmed/22534879. Accessed April 1, 2018.

9. Partridge ACR, Bai JW, Rosen CF, et al. Effectiveness of systemic treatments for Pyoderma gangrenosum: a systematic review of observational studies and clinical trials. Br J Dermatol 2018. https://doi.org/10.1111/bjd.16468. Available at: https://www.ncbi.nlm.nih.gov/pubmed/29451690. Accessed March 8, 2018.

10. Farhi D, Cosnes J, Zizi N, et al. Significance of erythema nodosum and pyoderma gangrenosum in inflammatory bowel diseases: a cohort study of 2402 patients. Medicine 2008;87(5):281–93. Available at: https://www.ncbi.nlm.nih.gov/pubmed/18794711. Accessed April 4, 2018.

11. DeFilippis EM, Feldman SR, Huang WW. The genetics of pyoderma gangrenosum and implications for treatment: a systematic review. Br J Dermatol 2014; 172(6):1487–97. Available at: https://onlinelibrary-wiley-com.libproxy.temple.edu/doi/full/10.1111/bjd.13493. Accessed March 10, 2018.

12. Kaffenberger BH, Trinidad J. Diagnosis uPGrade - Advances in pyoderma gangrenosum. JAMA Dermatol 2018. https://doi.org/10.1001/jamadermatol.2017.5979. Available at: https://jamanetwork.com/journals/jamadermatology/article-abstract/2672269?redirect=true. Accessed April 4, 2018.

13. Nasifoglu S, Heinrich B, Welzel J. Successful therapy of Pyoderma gangrenosum with a JAK2 inhibitor. Br J Dermatol 2018. https://doi.org/10.1111/bjd.16468. Available at: https://www.ncbi.nlm.nih.gov/pubmed/29451690. Accessed March 8 2018.

14. Koo K, Brem H, Lebwohl M. Pyoderma gangrenosum versus chronic venous ulceration: comparison of diagnostic features. J Cutan Med Surg 2006;10(1): 26–30. Available at: http://journals.sagepub.com.libproxy.temple.edu/doi/pdf/10.1007/7140.2006.00011. Accessed March 10, 2018.

Lower Limb Lymphedema

An Exploration of Various Treatment Methods

Adam Abboud, DPM, Jared Blum, DPM, Zarnab Butta, DPM,
Elizabeth Ferber Lindvig, DPM, Nishani Kuruppu, DPM,
Sonya Wali, DPM, Tracey C. Vlahovic, DPM*

KEYWORDS

- Lymphedema • Active exercise and compression therapy • Compression therapy

KEY POINTS

- Lower limb lymphedema impacts a patient's quality of life.
- Active exercise and compression therapy (AECT) has been shown to decrease limb volume and pain.
- Treatment goals are to maintain function, restore function, and decrease pain.

INTRODUCTION

Lymphedema is a progressive phenomenon in which fluid accumulates in tissue spaces, compromising lymphatic transport and leading to lymphatic system insufficiency.[1] More specifically, lower limb lymphedema (LLL) negatively impacts patients' mobility, physical strength, social activities, and psycho-emotional state. Patients with lymphedema experience pain from associated inflammation and ischemia, and primarily from the tissue distension from the accumulated lymph fluids.[1] If a patient with LLL is not properly treated, the condition will progress into further disability and a decline in quality of life.[2]

Primary forms of lymphedema occur in the absence of etiologic factors and are associated with congenital lymph vessel dysplasia and dysfunction. Primary lymphedema is difficult to diagnose during the early stages of development, which often delays patient care. Early initiation of therapy for lymphedema and strict compliance to therapeutic methods benefit the overall outcomes of lymphedema treatment in patients.[3] Several noninvasive and combination therapies have been researched to identify the success of different lymphedema treatment options. The therapies include compression therapy (CT), active exercise and compression (AECT), compression with liposuction, and compression with hypersaline diuretics. LLL can also result secondarily from other underlying etiologies in the body including injury, surgery, and neoplasm.

Temple University School of Podiatric Medicine, 148 North 8th Street, Philadelphia, PA 19107, USA
* Corresponding author.
E-mail address: traceyv@temple.edu

Clin Podiatr Med Surg 38 (2021) 589–593
https://doi.org/10.1016/j.cpm.2021.06.011
podiatric.theclinics.com

Lymphedema is frequently seen after traumatic injuries such as ankle and hindfoot fractures. This has a negative impact both preoperatively and postoperatively. Preoperatively, edema increases the time before surgical intervention can be performed. Postoperatively, edema can lead to various complications including wound complications and infection.[4] Because of this, various techniques have been developed with the goal of decreasing, stabilizing, or preventing edema.

Lymphaticovenular anastomosis (LVA) is a surgical intervention that can be performed on the contralateral limb when dealing with unilateral secondary LLL.[5] This article reviews therapy methods for both primary and secondary lymphedema currently available for LLL treatment.

PATIENT EVALUATION

A survey of lymphedema status in the lower extremity can be quantified using various parameters. These include limb volumes, body weight, performance status (Palliative Performance Scale), blood pressure, weakness, intensity of pain, laboratory tests, global distress score, intensity of pain, dyspnea, and weakness. Several methods for staging lymphedema have been developed and are not uniform across all studies.

Lymphedema staging is defined by the International Society of Lymphology (ISL) in 4 stages: stage 1, accumulation of tissue fluid, which is improved with limb elevation; stage 2, limb elevation alone is not enough to improve swelling, pitting is significant; stage 3, tissue appears hard and there is a lack of pitting, accompanying skin changes include thickening, hyperpigmentation, increased skin folds, fat deposits, and warty overgrowth.[6] Skin stiffness as a marker of lymphedema can be evaluated by palpation or pinching. Pitting edema can be evaluated by pressing on the skin for 5 seconds, with grades defined as such: 0, absence of pitting; 1, pitting present for $\leq$5s; 2, present for >5s.[1] Campsis Clinical Staging includes 5 stages of lymphedema assessment. Stage IA, no edema despite the presence of lymphatic dysfunction; stage IB, mild edema that spontaneously regresses with elevation; stage II, persistent edema that regresses only partially with elevation; stage III, persistent, progressive edema, recurrent erysipeloid lymphangitis; stage IV, fibrotic lymphedema with fibrotic limb; and stage V, elephantiasis with severe limb deformation.[7] These parameters were used by different studies as a measure of lymphedema and its regression due to treatment.

Nonpharmacologic Treatment Therapies

Lymphedema has been shown to be reduced significantly with the use of CT and active exercise. A study compared the efficacy of AECT therapy to CT alone. The study used multilayered compression bandaging with all participants, with compression pressure averaging around 64 mm Hg. In this study, AECT was performed with the patient bicycling with a resistance of 10% of maximum extension strength. Patients pedaled at a pace of 50 revolutions/min for 15 minutes. The CT-only patients maintained a seated position for 15 minutes. AECT and CT were shown to reduce lower limb volume by 62.5 $\pm$ 15.3% and 18.5 $\pm$ 15.0%, respectively.[1] Both methods reduced pain by 32.8% and 12%, respectively. Ultimately, AECT was shown to greatly improve LLL. CT alone was also shown to have some benefit in reducing gravitational influence, counteracting excessive leakage of blood vessels, and improving lymph propulsion and lymphatic drainage. Reduction in lower limb volume with AECT also reduced pain associated with tissue distension. Changes in skin stiffness and pitting were less remarkable between the 2 therapies, showing a little added benefit of exercise with CT.[1]

Lymphedema resulting from edematous patients undergoing surgical procedures not directly related to lymphedema is another area of treatment undergoing research. The standard method of treating edema is with ice and elevation. This has been shown to reduce preoperative edema (−5%) as well as limit edema postoperatively (+7%).[4] A newer strategy to combat edema is intermittent pulse CT, which applies pressure to the plantar arch to compress the local veins and lymphatic vessels to promote venous backflow. This has been shown to be ineffective in treating edema post-operatively (+46%) when supplementary techniques like elevation are not used.[4] One of the more effective methods to treat edema is the multilayer compression method, which has been shown to be more effective at reducing edema preoperatively (−23%) than ice with elevation. Also, although the ice and elevation method controls postoperative edema 2 days after intervention (+7%), this method has been shown to reduce post-operative edema in this time frame (−22%).[4]

Combination Therapies

Several combination therapies are being explored for the treatment of lymphedema. A viable option for lymphedema therapy includes a combination of CT with hypersaline diuretics. However, it is feasible only in cases that are refractory and in advanced disease state with patients who are resistant to diuretics alone.[6] A sample of 19 patients with advanced disease, such as cancer and congestive heart failure, were treated for bilateral pitting leg edema resistant to loop diuretic therapy. These patients were treated with combination limb compression and diuretics. CT included tubular stockinette and a synthetic padding, followed by layers of short-stretch bandages. Furosemide was administered over an hour in hypersaline IV solution and concurrently with compression, once a day.[6] Favorable results were noted after 3 days of therapy. A clinically significant decrease in limb volume was noted (decrease of 1.52 L) and the median weight loss in 15 patients was 3.1 kg. The values obtained from the patients indicated weight loss and reduction in fluid in both limbs.[6] The treatment was tolerated well by the patients, and stable levels of kidney profiles (creatinine clearance, sodium, potassium), blood pressure, and serum albumin were also noted.

Combination lymphedema treatment with both liposuction and CT resulted in the rapid decrease of excess fluid volume. The postoperative excess volume after 2 weeks was 1535 mL (reduction of 89%).[8] After liposuction and continuous CT, complete reduction was achieved 4 years after surgery and has lasted 11 years after initial treatment for the patient. The constant use of compression garments postoperatively played a major role in maintaining the result; the patient needed 2 compression garments every 2 months for the operated leg to keep the volume stable. The indications for liposuction included nonpitting swelling of the extremity and a lack of volume reduction by conservative regimens. The beneficial effects of liposuction are secondary to the removal of hypertrophied adipose tissue and increased blood flow in patients.[8] However, combination therapy with liposuction is proven most beneficial. In a 1989 study performed with patients with leg lymphedema, only an 8% reduction was reported in the group that underwent only liposuction.[9] The authors stated that because of the poor results, liposuction should mainly be used in arm lymphedema and if used for leg lymphedema, should be combined with excision or an alternative combination therapy. The combination therapy of preoperative CT and liposuction followed by postoperative CT led to a successful outcome in this patient; no recurrence of limb swelling was observed, due to continuous use and replacement of compression garments. In addition, no skin necrosis or cellulitis was observed. This study indicated that constant usage of compression garments is essential in maintaining size reduction.[8]

Surgical Treatments

In patients recovering from lower body neoplasms and cancer treatments, lymphedema can complicate and interfere with successful postoperative recovery. Subsequent lymphedema of the contralateral leg is a likely occurrence in patients who develop unilateral secondary LLL after the resection of gynecologic cancer. In some patients, even in an asymptomatic contralateral limb, there may be splash or stardust patterns present and seen with preoperative indocyanine green (ICG) fluorescent angiography.[5] The splash and stardust pattern is seen with lymphatic vessels undergoing retrograde flow, described by Yamamoto and colleagues, as a stage of lymphatic flow consistent with more severe forms of lymphedema.[8] LVA is a surgical intervention that can be performed on the contralateral limb when dealing with unilateral secondary LLL. This procedure may be a good option for preventative care in this patient population. A study performed by Onoda and colleagues followed up 10 patients for 6 months after the performance of a preventative minimally invasive LVA via a small incision.[10] Lymphatic ducts were marked preoperatively using ICG as well as subcutaneous veins using a vein viewer.[5] A 1 cm skin incision line was marked along the skin fold of the ankle where subcutaneous veins were close to lymph ducts.[5] Next a local anesthetic was administered, and an incision was made, and subcutaneous veins and lymph ducts were marked. Lymph ducts with viable lymphatic flow and large diameters were selected for anastomosis.[5] In cases where few veins were present compared with the number of lymph ducts, end-to-side anastomosis was performed on veins in addition to end-to-end anastomosis. After anastomosis, a patency test was performed, and the incision was closed. Patients were prescribed rest of both legs, IV antibiotics, and 1 week of vasodilators.[5]

The amount of reduction in lymphedema was assessed using the Campisi Clinical Staging at 2 weeks, 1 month, 3 months, and 6 months after surgery. At 6 months, 5 of the limbs that underwent preventative LVA procedure were at Campisi Clinical stage 0 and 5 were at Campisi Clinical stage 1A.[5]

Performing an LVA via a small incision at the ankle joint is ideal for 3 reasons. First geographically, it is a good location to spot and mark enough lymph ducts for the anastomosis to have a satisfactory outcome. Second, the incision in this region can be performed along the skin fold of the ankle, which leads to less noticeable scaring. Lastly, owing to its minimally invasive smaller incision, the operative period for the procedure is reduced as well. There was one case of postoperative lymphorrhea that was reported. This was due to leakage of lymphatic fluid from the proximal amputation stumps that were used for the LVA.[5] To rectify this, additional suturing was performed at the surgical site. In the future, it may be useful to anastomose the proximal lymph ducts with veins during lymph duct amputation. Furthermore, there is a need for a long-term follow-up with the 10 cases studied to monitor the progression of edema in these patients.[5]

SUMMARY

Lymphedema management and treatment is necessary to maintain and restore function to the lower limb. Patients seek treatment to decrease pain, social, and psychological struggle, as well as prevent the development of infection and further damage to the region because of poor lymphatic circulation. Because of the diverse causes of lymphedema, the therapies reviewed in this article examine nonpharmacologic therapies, combination therapies, and surgical therapy. Within nonpharmacologic therapies, CT with AECT was shown to be superior to CT alone. Although specific, tested therapies were deemed superior within different publications, none of the articles mentioned tested differences in efficacy among nonpharmacological, pharmacologic, and surgical options within a single comprehensive study; therefore, no single recommendation can be made as a gold standard treatment in LLL.

CLINICS CARE POINTS

- First, determine the cause of the lower limb lymphedema.
- Determine if the patient is a candidate for non-pharmacologic therapy such as AECT or CT.
- Upon follow up treatments, determine if patient is a candidate for surgical intervention or combination therapy.

DISCLOSURE

None of the authors have any financial interests to disclose for this article.

REFERENCES

1. Fukushima T, Tsuji T, Sano Y, et al. Immediate effects of active exercise with compression therapy on lower -limb lymphedema. J Support Care Cancer 2016;25:2603–10.
2. Finnane A, Hayes SC, Obermair A, et al. Quality of life of women with lower-limb lymphedema following gynecological. J Expert Rev Pharm Outcome Res 2011; 11:287–97.
3. Ogawa Y. Recent advancements in medical treatment for lymphedema. Ann Vasc Dis 2012;5(2):139–44.
4. Rohner-Spengler M, Frotzler A, Honigmann P, et al. Effective treatment of post-traumatic and postoperative edema in patients with ankle and hindfoot Fractures. The J Bone Joint Surg 2014;96(15):1263–71.
5. Onoda S, Todokoro T, Hara H, et al. Minimally invasive multiple lymphaticovenular anastomosis at the ankle for the prevention of lower leg lymphedema. Microsurgery 2016;34:372–6.
6. Gradalski T. Diuretics combined with compression in resistant limb edema of advanced disease - a case series report. J Pain Symptom Manage 2018;55(4): 1179–83.
7. Campisi C, Accogli S, Boccardo F. Lymphedema staging and surgical indications in geriatric age. BMC Geriatr 2010;10(suppl 1):A50.
8. Brorson H, Ohlin K, Olsson G, et al. Controlled compression and liposuction treatment for lower extremity lymphedema. Lymphology 2008;41:52–63.
9. Sando WC, Nahai F. Suction lipectomy in the management of limb lymphedema. Clin Plast Surg 1989;16:369–73.
10. Yamamoto T, Narushima M, Doi K, et al. Characteristic indocyanine green lymphography findings in lower extremity lymphedema: the generation of a novel lymphedema severity staging system using dermal backflow patterns. Plast Reconstr Surg 2011;127:1979–86.

Plantar Melanoma
An Investigation of Its Incidence

Michael An, DPM, Lev Blekher, DPM, Meng Liu, DPM,
Matthew Pitre, DPM, Ryan Shaner, DPM, Daryl Silva, DPM,
Tracey C. Vlahovic, DPM*

KEYWORDS

- Plantar • Melanoma • Incidence • Biopsy • Prevalence

KEY POINTS

- Acral Lenitginous Melanomas (ALM) often lack common features of classic melanoma. They may be amelanotic, or ulcerated, or may present as a wart.
- ALM has been associated with a worse prognosis compared with non-acral subtypes.
- It is imperative to get the diagnosis correct for ALM because misdiagnosing results in delay of treatment and a lower prognosis/patient outcome.

INTRODUCTION

Melanoma is a malignancy of the pigment producing melanocyte cells in the skin. The World Health Organization reports 132,000 cases of melanoma globally per year, while the American Cancer Association estimates 87,110 new cases in the United States in 2017.[1,2]

These cutaneous tumors can arise on any part of the skin, but range in frequency from 3% to 15% when they present on the foot and ankle.[3] Bristow and Bower[4] state that acral lentiginous melanoma (ALM) accounts for 60% of foot melanomas, with superficial spreading melanoma and nodular melanoma representing 40% and 9% of podiatric melanomas, respectively.[5,6]

ALMs often lack common features of classic melanoma. They may be amelanotic[4] or ulcerated[3,5] or may present as a wart.[7] Plantar melanoma also disproportionately afflicts African Americans and Asians,[8,9] even though melanoma in general is more commonly seen in whites.[2]

Lallas and colleagues[9] reported 99 plantar lesions suspect of melanoma were derived from retrospective data collected from 7 clinics in Austria, France, Japan, and Italy. Tas and Erturk[6] collected data from 1993 to 2015 from the Istanbul University Institute of Oncology and discovered 104 cases of plantar melanoma. Hui and colleagues[10] analyzed melanoma data from the central cancer registry of Hong Kong

Temple University School of Podiatric Medicine, 148 North 8th Street, Philadelphia, PA 19107, USA
* Corresponding author.
E-mail address: traceyv@temple.edu

from 1983 to 2002. The investigators discovered that 87% of melanoma occurring on the foot was present on plantar surfaces, in the data set examined.

However, no comprehensive data on the incidence of plantar melanoma explicitly exist for either the United States or on a global scale. As such, it would be of great benefit to the podiatric and general medical communities to investigate the frequency of plantar melanoma more thoroughly, especially when considering its predilection for minorities and its atypical features.

REVIEW OF THE LITERATURE

ALM has been associated with a worse prognosis compared with nonacral subtypes.[9] ALM accounts for 2% to 3% of all diagnosed melanomas, and it has a higher incidence in blacks and Hispanics than other types of melanomas. The worst survival rates were found in Hispanic populations and Asian Pacific Islanders.[11] ALM had thicker tumors when compared with other melanomas, and they were the thickest in women in the older decades of life. ALMs also have a significantly lower 10-year survival rate when compared with other malignant melanomas.[11]

ALM can mimic ulcerations, warts, onychomycosis, tinea pedis, subungual hematoma, vascular lesions, and infections, so there are several possible differential diagnoses to work up when diagnosing a patient with ALM. Having several possible differential diagnoses could be part of the reason up to one-third of cases of ALM are misdiagnosed. Half of the cases of ALM were found on the plantar surface of the foot, with the other half found interdigitally and subungually. Biopsy of an ALM sample is best done with an excisional, incisional, or punch biopsy rather than a shave biopsy due to its not encompassing the total depth of the tumor.[12]

An important demographic factor in the diagnosis of ALM is age of onset. According to Wolff and colleagues,[12] the median age of onset for ALM is 65 years. This age was similar to what was reported in Lallas and colleagues,[9] whereby the median age was 68 years with median age of men (66.5 years) slightly younger than women (71.1 years). However, Tsai and Chui[13] had a median age of 59 years for patients with plantar melanoma.[3] This discrepancy may be attributed to differences between sexes regarding ALM prevalence and ethnic differences regarding ALM diagnosis, respectively.

A scoring system for diagnosis of palmoplantar melanoma[14] was developed to reach the minimal specificity of 80%. According to Rubegni and colleagues,[14] cutaneous melanoma has a high prevalence in white populations, but the absolute incidence of acral melanoma is about the same across all races, with a significant portion of all cutaneous melanomas in non-white populations.[12] Rastrelli and colleagues[15] reports differ in that ALM accounts for 5% of melanomas in white patients but conclude similarly that ALM is the most common melanoma among Asian, Hispanic, and African patients. Wolff and colleagues[12] state similar incidences as Rastrelli (2014) with 2% to 8% ALM in whites and 50% ALM in ethnic groups.[11] A suggested reason for this trend was lack of awareness among patients about the presence of their ALM lesions. This lack of awareness increased the burden of diligence by the clinician to examine sites for pigmented lesions. Awareness of pigmented lesions increased when clinicians examined patients who presented for skin cancer-related visits as opposed to general dermatologic visits.[5] Tsai and Chui[13] reported that white patients were more likely to have undergone self-skin examination and full body skin examination by a health professional, but significant differences in reported ALM were not detected.

According to Wolff and colleagues,[12] ALM has a higher prevalence in men than in women at a ratio of 3:1.[11] Lallas and colleagues[9] reported the contrary with plantar melanoma having a higher prevalence in women with a male-to-female ratio of

1:1.6, but women often have a better prognosis. Tsai and Chui[13] also reported a higher female incidence, whereas Rastrelli and colleagues[15] and Tas and Erturk[6] reported elderly, female predominance regarding ALM diagnosis. This female predominance may be caused by shoe choices, as women are more likely to choose more fashionable but less comfortable shoes; however, more frequent foot problems lead to more frequent physician visits and potentially lead to early diagnosis and treatment of plantar melanoma. Plantar melanoma seems to follow the gait pattern, which is more likely to be on the lateral aspect of the heel and the ball of the foot, as weight-bearing is hypothesized to cause inflammation, which increases the risk of melanoma.[16]

AMELANOTIC AND SUBUNGUAL MELANOMAS AND THEIR INCIDENCE

There is a special type of plantar melanoma that presents as a nonhealing foot ulcer. It is usually undiagnosed or there is a delay in diagnosis.[17] Unlike the typical plantar melanoma, this type of melanoma may not present with discoloration or may be difficult to distinguish from a neuropathic plantar ulceration. In addition, a foot ulcer is commonly seen and rarely related to plantar melanoma as a differential diagnosis. Therefore, foot ulcers with unknown causations and chronic durations must be carefully evaluated, and a differential diagnosis of melanoma should be considered. A biopsy is important to diagnose this type of melanoma.[17]

Amelanotic melanoma can present as a hypopigmented form of any of the pigmented subtypes of cutaneous melanoma and is often confused for a variety of conditions.[18] When amelanotic melanoma appears on the plantar surface of the foot, it is likely a variation of ALM and often presents as a chronic lesion that does not heal with topical interventions. The misdiagnosis rate of all forms of acral melanoma has been cited as between 25% and 36%; however, this may be greater for acral amelanotic melanomas. Amelanotic melanoma constitutes 2% to 8% of all melanomas, but approximately 7% of amelanotic melanomas occurs on the plantar aspect of the foot.[19] These lesions may be painless to the patient and can at times resemble a diabetic foot ulcer.[20] Molecular studies have recently revealed that BRAF and NRAS mutations are common in melanomas that arise in areas without chronic sun-induced damage, such as the plantar aspect of the foot.[21] The molecular data indicated that KIT mutations occurred more readily in amelanotic acral melanomas versus pigmented acral melanomas: 12.1% versus 7.3%, respectively; thus the incidence of an amelanotic form of melanoma is greater in those with KIT mutations.[21]

Amelanotic forms of melanoma can occur on any part of the body and can fall under any subclassification of melanoma. In the case of plantar melanomas, approximately 7% are amelanotic in nature, and these lesions often resemble benign disorders, such as diabetic ulcers.[19] Histopathologic evidence of amelanosis was found in high incidence among the cases of aggressive melanoma, although the incidence of amelanosis was not found frequently among the cases described by Phan and colleagues.[8]

The atypical appearance of an amelanotic melanoma lesion often means that it is not identified until it reaches a more advanced stage than its pigmented counterpart. Improvements in dermoscopy have made the diagnosis of amelanotic melanoma easier, as dermoscopy currently allows for a sensitivity of 89% and a specificity of 96% in the diagnosis of amelanotic melanoma.[22] The dermoscopic approach to diagnosis relies on the clinician's ability to spot microvascular irregularities within the hypopigmented lesion, as these are telltale signs of melanoma despite hypopigmentation.[22]

In a study of the histopathology of ALM for incidence and prognostic features from 121 diagnosed cases, Phan and colleagues[8] found 15 cases of in situ melanoma, of which 13 were subungual. The other 106 cases were invasive ALM, with 9 at Clark level II, 35 at Clark level III, 40 at Clark level IV, and 22 at Clark level V. These cases were significantly associated with a high-mitotic rate and extensive ulceration, characteristics present in cases with severe invasion and poor outcomes.[8] Minimal or no pigment production was found in 34 of the cases. However, these lesions were associated with worse prognosis and increased tumor aggressiveness.[8]

Regarding factors not frequently associated with, or predictive of ALM, Phan and colleagues[8] found only 4 cases with cells suggestive of preexisting nevus lesions near the ALM lesions, of which 3 were at Clark level IV. Also, 99 of the 121 cases were in vertical growth phase, and many of these lesions were not associated with a high-mitotic rate.[8] Adnexal involvement was found in 56 of the ALM cases and was not associated with increased severity and therefore was deemed to have no prognostic value.[8]

SUMMARY

Ultimately, Phan and colleagues[8] found that increased ulceration and the associated high-mitotic rate, presence of microsatellites, and invasion at Clark level IV and V were in high incidence among the 121 cases of ALM. Thus, they determined these to be statistically significant prognostic factors in the time to recurrence and indicative of poor likelihood of survival.[8] Likewise, a mitotic rate greater than 6 mitoses per millimeter, as well as the presence of microsatellites, is predictive of high likelihood of metastasis and poor prognosis in ALM.[8] Last, increased metastasis, higher recurrence, and poorer prognosis were greater in men than in women among these 121 cases of ALM.[8]

Overall, plantar melanoma has a common range of absolute incidence among all races and is more prevalent in women. Inflammation is a potential risk factor of plantar melanoma. ALM usually does not stem from prior benign lesions, and the involvement of the deep dermis is not predictive of recurrence, although the incidence of such deep dermal involvement is a frequent clinical course.[8] Most importantly, it is imperative to get the diagnosis correct for ALM because misdiagnosing results in delay of treatment and a lower prognosis/patient outcome. There needs to be more emphasis in the future to the medical and podiatric communities of the proper diagnosis of plantar melanoma so melanoma patients can be properly treated in order to improve their overall outcome.

DISCLOSURE STATEMENT

None of the authors have any financial interests to disclose for this article.

REFERENCES

1. World Health Organization. How common is skin cancer 2017. Available at: http://www.who.int/uv/faq/skincancer/en/index1.html. Accessed March 6, 2018.
2. American Cancer Association. Cancer facts and figures 2017. Available at: https://www.cancer.org/research/cancer-facts-statistics/all-cancer-facts-figures/cancer-facts-figures-2017.html. Accessed March 6, 2018.
3. Bristow IR, de Berker DA, Acland KM, et al. Clinical guidelines for the recognition of melanoma of the foot and nail unit. J Foot Ankle Res 2010;3(25). https://doi.org/10.1186/1757-1146-3-25.
4. Bristow I, Bower C. Melanoma of the foot. Clin Podiatr Med Surg 2016;33:409–22.

5. Yin NC, Mteva M, Covington DS, Romanelli P, Stojadinovic O. The importance of wound biopsy in the accurate diagnosis of acral malignant melanoma presenting as a foot ulcer. Int J Lower Extremity Wounds 2013;12(4):289–92.
6. Tas F, Erturk K. Plantar melanoma is associated with certain poor prognostic histopathological factors, but not correlated with nodal involvement, recurrence, and worse survival. Clin Transl Oncol 2018;20(5):607–12.
7. De Giorgi V, Massi D. Images in clinical medicine. Plantar melanoma--a false vegetant wart. N Engl J Med 2006;355(13):e13. https://doi.org/10.1056/NEJMicm055674.
8. Phan A, Touzet S, Dalle S, et al. Acral lentiginous melanoma: histopathological prognostic features of 121 cases. Br J Dermatol 2007;157:311–8.
9. Lallas A, Sgouros D, Zalaudek I, et al. Palmar and plantar melanomas differ for sex prevalence and tumor thickness but not for dermoscopic patterns. Melanoma Res 2014;24(1):83–7.
10. Hui SK, Tang WYM, Wong TW, et al. Cutaneous melanoma: a population-based epidemiology report with 989 patients in Hong Kong. Clin Exp Dermatol 2007;32:265–7.
11. Swagata TA, Smita GS, Ashwini M, et al. Acral lentinginous melanoma: report of three cases. Egypt Dermatol Online J 2011;7(2):1–11, ser. 10.
12. Wolff K, Johnson RA, Saavedra AP, et al. Fitzpatrick's color atlas and synopsis of clinical dermatology. 8th edition. McGraw-Hill Education; 2017. Available at: https://accessmedicine.mhmedical.com/content.aspx?bookid=2043&sectionid=154893579. Accessed July 19, 2021.
13. Tsai MS, Chiu MW. Patient-reported frequency of acral surface inspection during skin examination in white and ethnic minority patients. J Am Acad Dermatol 2014;71(2):249–55.
14. Rubegni P, Cevenini G, Nami N, et al. A simple scoring system for the diagnosis of palmo-plantar pigmented skin lesions by digital dermoscopy analysis. J Eur Acad Dermatol Venereol 2013;e312–9.
15. Rastrelli M, Tropea S, Rossi CR, et al. Melanoma: epidemiology, risk factors, pathogenesis, diagnosis and classification. In Vivo 2014;28(6):1005–12.
16. Al-Hassani F, Chang C, Peach H. Acral lentiginous melanoma – is inflammation the missing link? JPRAS Open 2017;14:49–54.
17. Madankumar R, Gumaste PV, Martires K, et al. Acral melanocytic lesions in the United States: prevalence, awareness, and dermoscopic patterns in skin-of-color and non-Hispanic white patients. J Am Acad Dermatol 2016;74(4):724–30.e1.
18. Patel KA, Ferraro AJ. Acral lentiginous melanoma: a case and literature review. Foot Ankle Online J 2015;8(1):1, ser. 1.
19. Koch SE, Lange JR. Amelanotic melanoma: the great masquerader. J Am Acad Dermatol 2000;42(5):731–4.
20. Yesil S, Demir T, Akinci B, et al. Amelanotic melanoma misdiagnosed as a diabetic foot ulcer. J Diabetes Complications 2007;21:335–7.
21. Kim JK, Lee J, Kim S, et al. Amelanotic acral melanoma associated with KIT mutation and vitiligo. Ann Dermatol 2015;27(2):201–5.
22. Stoecker WV, Stolz W. Dermoscopy and the diagnostic challenge of amelanotic and hypomelanotic melanoma. Arch Dermatol 2008;144(9):1207–10.

UNITED STATES POSTAL SERVICE ®

Statement of Ownership, Management, and Circulation
(All Periodicals Publications Except Requester Publications)

1. Publication Title	2. Publication Number	3. Filing Date
CLINICS IN PODIATRIC MEDICINE & SURGERY	000 – 707	9/18/2021

4. Issue Frequency	5. Number of Issues Published Annually	6. Annual Subscription Price
JAN, APR, JUL, OCT	4	$310.00

7. Complete Mailing Address of Known Office of Publication (Not printer) (Street, city, county, state, and ZIP+4®)

ELSEVIER INC.
230 Park Avenue, Suite 800
New York, NY 10169

Contact Person
Malathi Samayan

Telephone (Include area code)
91-44-4299-4507

8. Complete Mailing Address of Headquarters or General Business Office of Publisher (Not printer)

ELSEVIER INC.
230 Park Avenue, Suite 800
New York, NY 10169

9. Full Names and Complete Mailing Addresses of Publisher, Editor, and Managing Editor (Do not leave blank)

Publisher (Name and complete mailing address)

DOLORES MELONI, ELSEVIER INC.
1600 JOHN F KENNEDY BLVD. SUITE 1800
PHILADELPHIA, PA 19103-2899

Editor (Name and complete mailing address)

LAUREN BOYLE, ELSEVIER INC.
1600 JOHN F KENNEDY BLVD. SUITE 1800
PHILADELPHIA, PA 19103-2899

Managing Editor (Name and complete mailing address)

PATRICK MANLEY, ELSEVIER INC.
1600 JOHN F KENNEDY BLVD. SUITE 1800
PHILADELPHIA, PA 19103-2899

10. Owner (Do not leave blank. If the publication is owned by a corporation, give the name and address of the corporation immediately followed by the names and addresses of all stockholders owning or holding 1 percent or more of the total amount of stock. If not owned by a corporation, give the names and addresses of the individual owners. If owned by a partnership or other unincorporated firm, give its name and address as well as those of each individual owner. If the publication is published by a nonprofit organization, give its name and address.)

Full Name	Complete Mailing Address
WHOLLY OWNED SUBSIDIARY OF REED/ELSEVIER, US HOLDINGS	1600 JOHN F KENNEDY BLVD. SUITE 1800 PHILADELPHIA, PA 19103-2899

11. Known Bondholders, Mortgagees, and Other Security Holders Owning or Holding 1 Percent or More of Total Amount of Bonds, Mortgages, or Other Securities. If none, check box ☐ None

Full Name	Complete Mailing Address
N/A	

12. Tax Status (For completion by nonprofit organizations authorized to mail at nonprofit rates) (Check one)
The purpose, function, and nonprofit status of this organization and the exempt status for federal income tax purposes:
☒ Has Not Changed During Preceding 12 Months
☐ Has Changed During Preceding 12 Months (Publisher must submit explanation of change with this statement)

PS Form 3526, July 2014 [Page 1 of 4 (see instructions page 4)] PSN: 7530-01-000-9931 PRIVACY NOTICE: See our privacy policy on www.usps.com

13. Publication Title			14. Issue Date for Circulation Data Below
CLINICS IN PODIATRIC MEDICINE & SURGERY			JULY 2021

15. Extent and Nature of Circulation			Average No. Copies Each Issue During Preceding 12 Months	No. Copies of Single Issue Published Nearest to Filing Date
a. Total Number of Copies (Net press run)			163	149
b. Paid Circulation (By Mail and Outside the Mail)	(1)	Mailed Outside-County Paid Subscriptions Stated on PS Form 3541 (Include paid distribution above nominal rate, advertiser's proof copies, and exchange copies)	100	91
	(2)	Mailed In-County Paid Subscriptions Stated on PS Form 3541 (Include paid distribution above nominal rate, advertiser's proof copies, and exchange copies)	0	0
	(3)	Paid Distribution Outside the Mails Including Sales Through Dealers and Carriers, Street Vendors, Counter Sales, and Other Paid Distribution Outside USPS®	13	11
	(4)	Paid Distribution by Other Classes of Mail Through the USPS (e.g. First-Class Mail®)	0	0
c. Total Paid Distribution (Sum of 15b (1), (2), (3), and (4))			113	102
d. Free or Nominal Rate Distribution (By Mail and Outside the Mail)	(1)	Free or Nominal Rate Outside-County Copies included on PS Form 3541	34	31
	(2)	Free or Nominal Rate In-County Copies Included on PS Form 3541	0	0
	(3)	Free or Nominal Rate Copies Mailed at Other Classes Through the USPS (e.g. First-Class Mail)	0	0
	(4)	Free or Nominal Rate Distribution Outside the Mail (Carriers or other means)	0	0
e. Total Free or Nominal Rate Distribution (Sum of 15d (1), (2), (3) and (4))			34	31
f. Total Distribution (Sum of 15c and 15e)			147	133
g. Copies not Distributed (See Instructions to Publishers #4 (page #3))			16	16
h. Total (Sum of 15f and g)			163	149
i. Percent Paid (15c divided by 15f times 100)			76.87%	76.69%

* If you are claiming electronic copies, go to line 16 on page 3. If you are not claiming electronic copies, skip to line 17 on page 3.

16. Electronic Copy Circulation		Average No. Copies Each Issue During Preceding 12 Months	No. Copies of Single Issue Published Nearest to Filing Date
a. Paid Electronic Copies	▲		
b. Total Paid Print Copies (Line 15c) + Paid Electronic Copies (Line 16a)	▲		
c. Total Print Distribution (Line 15f) + Paid Electronic Copies (Line 16a)	▲		
d. Percent Paid (Both Print & Electronic Copies) (16b divided by 16c × 100)	▲		

☒ I certify that 50% of all my distributed copies (electronic and print) are paid above a nominal price.

17. Publication of Statement of Ownership

☒ If the publication is a general publication, publication of this statement is required. Will be printed in the OCTOBER 2021 issue of this publication. ☐ Publication not required.

18. Signature and Title of Editor, Publisher, Business Manager, or Owner	Date
Malathi Samayan - Distribution Controller *Malathi Samayan*	9/18/2021

I certify that all information furnished on this form is true and complete. I understand that anyone who furnishes false or misleading information on this form or who omits material or information requested on the form may be subject to criminal sanctions (including fines and imprisonment) and/or civil sanctions (including civil penalties).

PS Form 3526, July 2014 (Page 3 of 4) PRIVACY NOTICE: See our privacy policy on www.usps.com

Moving?

Make sure your subscription moves with you!

To notify us of your new address, find your **Clinics Account Number** (located on your mailing label above your name), and contact customer service at:

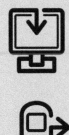

Email: journalscustomerservice-usa@elsevier.com

800-654-2452 (subscribers in the U.S. & Canada)
314-447-8871 (subscribers outside of the U.S. & Canada)

Fax number: 314-447-8029

Elsevier Health Sciences Division
Subscription Customer Service
3251 Riverport Lane
Maryland Heights, MO 63043

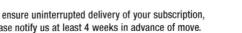